Tired of not ꞌ ꞌꞁeping?

A COMPLETE & PRACTICAL GUIDE TO OVERCOMING INSOMNIA

By Sandra Cabot MD and Nancy Beckham ND

Tired of not Sleeping?
Copyright © 2005 Sandra Cabot MD & Nancy Beckham ND

Published by

SCB International Inc.
PO Box 5070 Glendale AZ USA 85312
Phone 623 334 3232

www.liverdoctor.com
www.weightcontroldoctor.com

ISBN: 978-09757436-0-7

1) Sleep 2) Insomnia 3) Depression 4) Anxiety

Contents

About the Authors

Dr Sandra Cabot MBBS, DRCOG, is a medical doctor who has extensive clinical experience; she treats patients with hormonal imbalances, chronic diseases and weight problems.

Her practices are situated in Camden and Sydney, NSW Australia. Dr Sandra Cabot began studying nutritional medicine while she was a medical student and has been a pioneer in the area of holistic healing. She graduated in medicine with honours from the University of Adelaide, South Australia in 1975. During the 1980s Dr Cabot worked as a volunteer in the largest missionary Christian hospital in India, tending to the poor indigenous women.

Dr Cabot founded the National Health Advisory Service in 1981, as a non-government funded service. This service has provided telephone and internet advice for people of all ages who want to know all their options.

For more information phone Dr Cabot's Health Line on 623 344 3232 in the USA and 02 4655 8855 in Australia.

Dr Cabot pilots herself to many cities and country towns in Australia where she is invited to speak at seminars and exhibitions.

For further information about Dr Sandra Cabot read on line at www.weightcontroldoctor.com and www.liverdoctor.com

---

Nancy Beckham is a naturopath, herbalist, homeopath and yoga teacher. At 43 years of age Nancy developed serious health problems and embarked on a self help program that was so successful it enabled her to avoid a proposed hip replacement and anti-inflammatory drugs; this lead to her decision to become a natural therapist.

Nancy has 25 years of experience as a natural therapy practitioner and has run workshops and seminars for the general public and practitioners. Nancy is also an academic and researcher, and has written several books including: *Heart & Circulation, The Family Guide to Natural Therapies, The Australian Guide to Natural Therapies, Menopause - a positive approach using natural therapies, Menopause & Osteoporosis and Rejuvenation.*

Introduction

Most humans enjoy sleeping and you often hear people say 'I had a great sleep' even though they were not conscious of sleeping. Sleep is basically a restorative process for your body, your mind and perhaps your Spirit. During the day you rely on other people for various things but while sleeping you are self-sufficient, and at the same time you have a break from your personal problems and the problems of the world.

Not being able to sleep is distressing. Thoughts seem to be racing around the brain or one thought is continuous, and the body is restless. The more you *try* to sleep the more agitated you become. The more you worry, think and talk about sleep the more sleep eludes you.

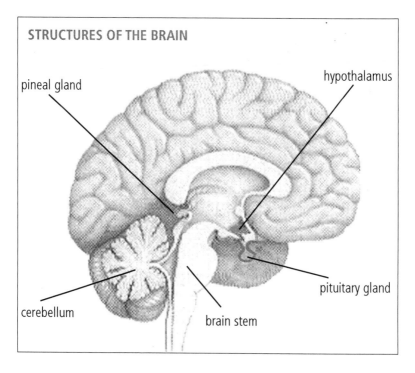

STRUCTURES OF THE BRAIN

pineal gland

hypothalamus

pituitary gland

cerebellum

brain stem

Signs of insomnia include trouble falling asleep, waking during the night, waking up very early and not getting back to sleep, and non-restorative sleep. Insomnia is often accompanied by reduced functioning during the day, fatigue, poor concentration and memory, not coping with even minor irritations, and general lack of motivation or enjoyment.

THE DIFFERENT TYPES OF INSOMNIA

The broad categories of sleep disorders are given below:

- **Transient (temporary) insomnia** may last a week or so and is linked to changes such as a new job or an overseas trip.

- **Short-term insomnia** is when sleep is disrupted for a few months and may be triggered by a stressful event, such as job loss or a serious illness.

- **Chronic or long-term insomnia** is a problem with the quality or amount of sleep you get and is defined as persisting for more than a few months. Severe or prolonged insomnia may affect between 20 — 30 per cent of adults.

- **Secondary insomnia** is when sleep is diminished because of something else such as pain or inappropriate drug intake.

- **Primary insomnia** includes disorders of the body's sleep clock and sleep apnoea.

  Humans have an internal biological sleep clock that controls the sleep-wake cycle (see diagram on page 11). This inner clock is located within the hypothalamus — the part of the brain that also controls hormones, body temperature, thirst and appetite. The primary sleep clock in the brain is modulated by the natural light cycle but is also affected by genes and by many environmental, biochemical and lifestyle factors.

  The word apnoea means 'without breath' and some people actually stop breathing for short periods of time during sleep. Symptoms of sleep apnoea include loud snoring, together with choking or gasping episodes during sleep and daytime fatigue.

- **Idiopathic insomnia** simply means that a cause has not been identified.

•**Pseudoinsomnia** is when people believe they have insomnia but they actually sleep quite well. For example, an elderly person who goes to bed around 9 p.m. and wakes at 4 a.m. has probably had enough sleep! Some think they should fall asleep a few minutes after they get into bed while others believe that they have long periods of wakefulness during the night. You may believe that you lie awake for hours but this may not be the reality because you're not conscious of sleeping during deep sleep. Pseudoinsomnia can progress to real insomnia because worrying sleep messages are being sent to the brain. An important message in this book is that too much thinking about sleep can lead to insomnia.

The Hypothalamus and the body functions it controls and regulates

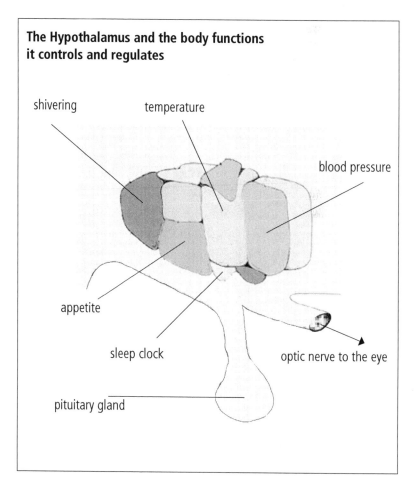

shivering

temperature

blood pressure

appetite

sleep clock

optic nerve to the eye

pituitary gland

SLEEP PROBLEMS

I think the world is divided into good sleepers and poor sleepers — and poor sleepers are very sensitive to any type of change or stress. Good sleepers can usually sleep anywhere and are known to be able to "sleep on a barbed wire fence"! Women are said to absorb more 'cues' from the environment and this may explain why they have more sleep problems than men.

When you are about to sleep you may experience muscle jerking or a falling sensation and this is called 'sleep starts' and is considered normal. Disorders, such as sleep talking or mild snoring, usually do not require treatment although there may be causes such as stress, upper respiratory tract problems or unhealthy lifestyle habits.

Sleep deprivation may be a choice. Some complain that they feel tired during the day but they're attached to staying up late at night, perhaps to enjoy relaxation or freedom. Whole families may be deprived of sleep because the evening meal is delayed for various reasons, or they have stimulating evening activities that overpower the inclination to sleep. Others may have bed resistance, which simply means that they don't like going to bed.

As you will see in Chapter 3, there are many causes of insomnia. For instance, modern lifestyles may suit some people but be exhausting, over-stimulatory or stressful for others. However, insomnia is not only a problem of our technological age. Prehistoric people probably had sleeping problems due to physical discomforts, hunger, violence and fears.

Our known ancestors certainly had sleep problems, as you will see from literature, history books and the Bible.

When I lie down, I think, 'When will it be day that I may rise?'
When the evening grows long and I lie down,
I do nothing but toss till morning twilight.
Job 7.4

In my clinical experience, most insomniacs have anxious person-
alities and this is confirmed by tests showing that insomniacs tend
to have higher levels of adrenal gland stress hormones (cortisol
and adrenalin) compared to good sleepers. You can't avoid
stress, but you can modify the way you handle stress and you can
change the way you think and react.

If you are feeling well in spite of getting somewhat less sleep
than average, don't worry about this. However, if your sleep time
is well below the average of seven hours you might consider
gradually adjusting your sleeping habits because this may improve
your wellbeing, and marginal sleep deprivation may contribute to
health problems as you age.

NORMAL SLEEP

Healthful sleep is a variable process that progresses from a short,
drowsy phase to deeper restorative stages where the brain waves
slow down. Within the slow wave stages there are periods of
rapid eye movement (REM) sleep when the brain waves are more
active and this is when most dreaming occurs. During REM sleep
the heart rate increases — as if you were acting out the dream.
A cycle of slow wave and REM sleep typically lasts 90 — 120
minutes with 4 — 5 cycles each night. As the night progresses,
there is relatively more active REM sleep compared to slow wave
sleep and these varied sleep processes affect different parts of the
brain, and the different parts of the brain communicate with each
other. As daylight approaches you revert back to lighter stages of
slow wave sleep.

When you sleep your brain is processing your daily activities
and doing homework for you; it doesn't actually need your
conscious help but needs your cooperation to leave it alone to
get the job done. Appropriate amounts of both REM sleep and

non-REM (slow wave) sleep are required to keep you mentally balanced because the left and right hemispheres of your brain are alternatively activated at different sleep stages. You feel much better if you sleep well and this is because your nervous system, organs, immune system, hormones and cells get a break from daily demands.

HOW TO USE THIS BOOK

My recommendation is to minimise thinking about sleep (except for working out a few healthful strategies) and *not* to analyse how you slept when you wake in the morning. In other words, *do* something rather than dwelling on the problem.

- Have a quick skim through the whole book to familiarise yourself with the contents. Then ask yourself if you really have a sleeping problem, given that individual needs for sleep vary widely. Your judgement should be based on how you *usually* sleep because we are all upset at times due to the ups and downs of everyday life. Perhaps your insomnia is a secondary effect of some other problem, such as pain, in which case the cause should be found and treated.

- Look at the list of causes in Chapter 3 and see if there are any simple steps that you can take to improve your sleep.

- Make a judgement about your best insomnia treatment options. Your options might include early morning outdoor exercise in the sunlight, aromatherapy, a relaxation tape, magnesium tablets, homeopathic remedies or a herbal remedy.

- For many insomniacs there is not *one* single cause and that's why I recommend trying a few (say 2 to 3) strategies at a time. If you try too many strategies and remedies all at once this may increase agitation and stress.

For people with long-term insomnia, my initial treatment usually includes what I call 'diversion therapy'. Do not try too hard, because this gives your brain multiple sleep messages that may cause even more anxiety about sleep. Remember, sleep is instinctive and not a mental process — and the primary purpose of human life (and sleep) is to enjoy it!

Insomniacs are often advised not to sleep or nap during the day. However, in some sleep deprivation cases, short naps may improve wellbeing, reduce heart disease and improve learning.[1] Naps should be less than 30 minutes to avoid awakening from deep sleep and then not being sufficiently alert to function safely. Shift workers are likely to benefit from a short nap at work (although I doubt that this is an option that most employers allow), and naps may also help mothers and carers who have interrupted nighttime sleep.

Avoid talking about your insomnia, (except with your health practitioner) because this not only gives your mind insomnia messages but may also trigger a problem in other people, or set yourself up to get confusing and irritating advice from people who sleep well. I'm sure you know people who drink coffee late at night and do all the wrong things and yet they sleep beautifully but the mere smell of coffee may keep an insomniac awake until 4 a.m.

Finding and removing the cause of sleep problems is rarely simple because a number of causes may be present at the same time. Individuals who are sensitive to noise, light and temperature may also overreact to work and relationship stresses — and insomnia further reduces emotional and mental vigor.

For all health problems, if your own efforts are not successful, consult a practitioner. This book discusses the use of antidepressant drugs and sleeping pills, because we want to provide you with a holistic approach to a difficult problem. Sleeping pills should be used as a last resort and for short periods in cases of stress overload, grief and trauma.

If you have a health problem do something about it now because it may not go away by itself and indeed may very well get worse. This book will inspire you, inform you and guide you and you can trust its advice, as it is based upon the collective knowledge of two very well known, respected and highly experienced health practitioners.

Chapter 1

SLEEP REQUIREMENTS

Be aware of the individuality of sleep: Some need more sleep than others to function efficiently; some sleep readily and wake refreshed under almost any conditions while others are easily disturbed.

If you lie in bed 'longing for sleep' your perception of time may not be realistic and some self-diagnosed insomniacs actually underestimate sleeping time.[1] In other words, when you say 'I lie awake for hours every night' the time awake may actually be only 20 or 30 minutes. You don't remember anything while in deep sleep and it is possible that your memory may only be aware of your waking episodes. Of course, it's preferable to sleep through the night.

HOW MUCH SLEEP DO YOU NEED?

Sleep experts do not agree on sleep requirements. Some are reverting to the recommendation that we need eight hours of sleep a night while most recommend between 5 — 9 hours for adults. A few suggest that 'normal' adult sleep requirements vary from 3 — 10 hours, with a caution that insufficient sleep may lead to illness.

You may have heard prominent people boasting how they function on only a few hours' sleep a night; however, you don't know if their decision-making has been impaired, or had they slept longer perhaps conflicts and even wars may have been averted. How do these 'short sleepers' relate to their colleagues and their families? Have 'short sleepers' equally short tempers, have they relationship or communication problems, and will they eventually experience health consequences? When people are in public they are probably on their best behavior, so *you* don't know how they are feeling and behaving most of the time.

Accidents are often caused by sleep problems due to dulled reflexes, mental lapses, irritability and impatience — and that's why you need quality sleep. Although you may become accustomed to sleep deprivation, you may not be aware that long-term sleep restriction results in reduced mental functioning.[2] It is highly likely that *more* sleep may make you more energetic, happier and smarter.

AVERAGE SLEEP PER DAY

Babies normally sleep between 16 to 20 hours, young teenagers about nine hours, and the average for an adult is about seven hours, although during pregnancy women often need one to two hours more than usual. After age 60, average sleep is about 6 ½ hours. Research indicates that 100 years ago adults in developed countries were averaging nine hours sleep a night, so it is possible that in today's hectic world many of us are actually sleep deprived.

SLEEP ONSET

The average adult takes 15 to 20 minutes to get to sleep. Some researchers suggest that if you fall asleep within five minutes this may be a sign of sleep deprivation but I think this may be normal for some lucky people and it often happens when you have had unusual or extra physical activity. Perhaps adults need a little quiet reflective time before sleep? Before puberty, children generally fall asleep within 10 minutes.

If you routinely take more than 30 minutes to fall asleep, you may need to change some aspects of your lifestyle, use stress management techniques or a longer wind down period before bed — or you may have insomnia if this is coupled with poor functioning during the day.

Some people are 'owls' (evening types) while others are 'larks' (morning types) and this indicates that individual biological sleep clocks are set differently, although the clocks can be modified. The larks are asleep by about 9 to 10 p.m. and wake feeling lively at 5 to 6 a.m. The owls love staying up late, *preferring* to get up after 7.30 a.m. and if they are functioning well, this is not a problem if it ties in with work, family and social commitments. Some owls are grumpy for the first few hours of the day but they are usually okay around mid-morning and peak after dinner. Work, school, family and social life may not tie in with the natural sleeping pattern of many owls because today's daily routines are largely geared to larks.

Sleep requirements are individual and some adults function more effectively if they have nine hours sleep, while others apparently manage very well on five hours. If *you* are not functioning well, the cause may be insufficient sleep, non-restorative sleep and occasionally too much sleep.

SLEEP MAINTENANCE

If you wake during most nights and it takes you more than 30 minutes to get back to sleep, you have insomnia — and the cause should be investigated. Fragmented sleep means that you have more light sleep relative to restorative deep sleep.

As a general guideline, about 85 per cent of your time in bed should be spent sleeping. It is often said that you should get up and do something if you can't sleep, but you are often too groggy to get out of bed — and you *want* to sleep and you want to feel lively the next day. Also, if you get up and start doing something in the middle of the night this means turning on lights and your brain will think it's morning — further disrupting your biological sleep clock and stopping production of melatonin (your sleep hormone).

My suggestion is to use audio books or disks and instead of *trying* to sleep you can lie in the dark focusing on the words or the meaning. In Chapter 3 under 'sleep routine insufficiency' I give some suggestions about the types of audio books and tapes that may be helpful. This is a useful activity that you can do in the dark and is not too stimulating. I find that the more I tell myself to listen to every word, the quicker I get back to sleep. Some insomniacs find that listening to the radio or soft music is comforting and sends them back to sleep. However, if nothing works, it's better to be doing something rather than lying in bed annoying yourself. Some insomniacs have interesting or useful hobbies. An obvious choice is to study a new subject or course that you have always wanted to pursue but never had time for. You could also take up astronomy; you can buy maps and telescopes or at least learn the constellations that you can see with the naked eye. There are so many interesting and useful things to learn and do.

Some people apparently adapt to limited night sleep, plus naps throughout the day, and this may provide relief for mothers with young children, carers and shift workers.

WAKING UP IN THE MORNING

Waking very early following less than six hours sleep may also be a form of insomnia — if you have problems with daytime functioning. Others wake in a 'twilight zone' and lie in bed half-asleep and half-awake for more than 30 minutes. If getting out of bed is a problem, you might try more fresh air in the bedroom, fewer bedcovers, allowing a little early morning light into the bedroom, or setting the alarm so you restrict the time you lie in bed *not* sleeping. Give yourself a reward for getting out of bed; perhaps a cup of freshly ground coffee and an outdoor walk. Early morning is very pleasant once you get used to it!

Most people function better if they have a *regular* pattern of sleeping. For instance, if you 'sleep in' on Sunday, you may not feel sleepy until relatively late that evening — and consequently Monday is a not a good day because you are sleep deprived. Although sleeping in on the weekends may worsen insomnia, you have to offset this against the pleasurable effects of *not* getting out of bed, being able to relax and not being fanatical about routine. An option for insomniacs is to get up and have a delicious, leisurely breakfast — outside if the weather permits, or listen to your favorite music while doing some energizing stretches. In other words, have your relaxation and break from the routine out of bed.

IDEAL SLEEPING TIME-ZONE

It is commonly agreed that the ideal sleeping time zone for an adult to regenerate their best level of physical and mental health is between 10 p.m. and 6 a.m. This time zone of 10 p.m. to 6 a.m. coincides with biological re-balancing changes such as core body temperature and hormone levels. In order to get uninterrupted sleep, you may need to be asleep about 6 — 8 hours before your lowest body temperature is reached, otherwise your brain may wake you to let you know you are getting cold. The temperature factor is a disadvantage of going to bed late and a number of my patients say they wake about 5.00 a.m. because they feel cold. Overheating can also greatly disrupt sleep and the relationship between temperature and sleep is covered in Chapter 3.

ADOLESCENT SLEEP

A 1980 sleep laboratory study indicated that adolescents require *more* sleep than pre-teens.[3] At thirteen years of age about ten hours sleep may be required, however, many at this age get less — and this sleep deprivation may lead to reduced immune function, daytime fatigue and *mood swings*.

Researchers suggest that at puberty the biological sleep clock is reset and the changing body produces signals to go to bed later and get up later, however, the problem is that this does not coincide with household and school routines.

Of course, at puberty young people want to be independent and socially active, and going to bed at 'kid's time' is not appealing. You may be able to explain to them that their additional sleep needs are temporary because they are changing from being a kid to being an adult. Entice them to go to bed earlier, in fifteen-minute steps, by preparing a small, tasty bedtime snack. Another option, if practicable, is to allow them to get up slightly later in the mornings. Encourage sports and physical activity, perhaps with *subtle* reminders of the training regimes of sports heroes.

Young people also have varying sleep needs and a specific number of hours only become relevant if there is persistent sleepiness during the day or excessive mood swings. I've found in my yoga classes that some adults like listening to stories for relaxation, so you might try reading to teenagers at bedtime. Select something non-stimulating and appropriate to their interests (such as biographies of sports stars or stories of explorers) and don't tell their friends about the bedtime reading!

SLEEP IN THE ELDERLY

You may think that when you retire you'll be able to sleep in. The irony is that when you, at last, have more time, you actually have somewhat reduced sleeping quality and capacity. Not only does stage three and four slow wave sleep decline with age but also various factors tend to wake you during the night, such as bladder and joint disorders. You may find that a sensible strategy is to have more interests rather than vainly attempting to get more sleep.

You don't need an expert to tell you that older people tend to get sleepy earlier in the evening and they wake earlier compared to young adults. The cycles of body temperature and production of the sleep hormone melatonin advance by about one hour in people aged between 65 — 75 years.[4]

Given that the average sleeping time in those aged over 60 years is about 6½ hours, it is obvious that if you go to bed at 9 p.m. and are asleep by, say, 9.30 p.m. you may have had enough sleep around 4.30 a.m. Generally, it is not healthy to lie in bed awake for long periods of time because this may weaken you physically, and upset your biological sleep clock. Lying in bed for hours in a state somewhere between sleep and wakefulness, tends to make you feel tired when you finally get out of bed, and it may be fine to do this occasionally as a treat but not as a routine habit.

As a general rule, if you sleep around 6½ hours you should not spend more than one additional hour in bed, as this is not good for your bones, joints, muscles and circulation, as well as giving your brain the message that your bed is for frustration and worry.

This typical sleeping duration in older people leaves around 17½ hours for daily activity, including some relaxation. Many elderly people complain to their doctors that they wake up very early and can't get back to sleep, and consequently they are prescribed sleeping pills instead of reality advice.

A problem in the elderly is that if they get up earlier and earlier, their exposure to early morning light, particularly in the summer, tends to reinforce earlier evening sleepiness. One solution may be to get out of bed soon after waking, keep the blinds and curtains closed, have dim lighting — and meditate in a sitting position. Prepare your meditation area the night before, keep the house uncluttered and safe in order to prevent falls and injuries in the dim early morning light. Then get outdoor light exposure.

Activities in the evening, starting just before the normal bedtime, may shift the sleeping pattern so that, if desired, older people may change their biological sleep clocks and be able to go to bed later and get up later. The activities might include walking, tai chi, gentle yoga, or an exercise bike. Bright evening light, socializing, playing cards, learning something new and timed melatonin supplementation may also help shift nighttime sleepiness to somewhat later times.

A controlled-release melatonin product improved sleep efficiency in elderly people.[5] The beneficial use of melatonin supplementation has been confirmed in a number of studies and further details about melatonin supplements are given in Chapter 5.

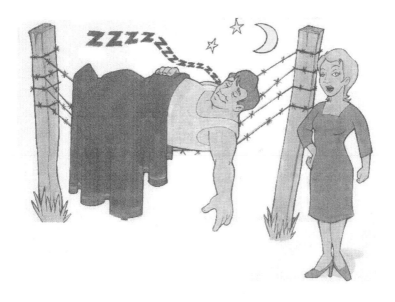

Some lucky people can sleep anywhere. . . .
Even on a barbed wire fence!!

Chapter 2

WHY YOU NEED A GOOD NIGHT'S SLEEP

The benefits of adequate and restorative sleep include:

- •Optimizing daytime physical performance
- •Optimizing daytime mental performance (improved learning, memory and concentration)
- •Preventing injuries and accidents
- •Slowing down the ageing process and a longer life span because of rest, repair and reduced oxidation
- •Improving immune function
- •Improving metabolism and some studies have shown that sleep deprivation increases the tendency to being overweight
- •Helping to maintain wellbeing, happiness and good relationships
- •Reducing 'sickies' and therefore contributing to the economy
- •Providing respite from your daily problems and your conscious mind

MENTAL AND PHYSICAL PERFORMANCE

It is said that a sleeping brain is a learning brain because that's when your learning is consolidated. After a visual discrimination test, improvement in performance was not observed unless there had been at least six hours of sleep prior to retesting

Whatever the mechanism, the sleeping brain appears to be doing some re-learning for you and, getting to sleep relatively early at night seems to give extra enhancement to memory and learning.[2]

Physically we need rest for cell regeneration and to allow the body to detoxify. For instance, if you are constantly active you get a build-up of lactic acid that causes muscle pain as well as anxiety.

Human sleep laboratory experiments confirm that different stages of sleep are linked to different types of memory experiences and that different parts of the brain are involved. A complete sleep is known to improve the ability to learn languages, to improve visual recognition, to improve mathematical problem solving and to consolidate motor skills such as playing a musical instrument and typing.

Most of us experience for ourselves that after a bad night's sleep we have less motivation, patience and energy for physical and mental activities. You may think you are okay with minimal sleep but you are actually incurring a 'sleep debt' and your judgement and functioning are at least subtly impaired. When you hear someone boasting about how they work through the night, you might wonder if healthful sleep would make them happier and more accomplished.

ACCIDENTS

Sleep deprivation is a potent cause of motor vehicle accidents, as well as many other types of accidents, and there are various obvious explanations for this. A less known reason is that your usual visual field deteriorates with lack of sleep so that there is less ability to process what is happening around you.[3] This particular deficit means that sideways vision is reduced but you may not realize this because it is a partial impairment. (You may have experienced for yourself that if you have a standard eye test when you are exhausted your test results are poor compared to when you are feeling well.)

A number of people have sleep inadequacies that cause 'microsleeps' during the day but they may not be aware of this fleeting loss of consciousness. Lack of sleep seems to coincide with a general lack of awareness. A decrease in sleep of about

1.5 hours can reduce daytime alertness by 33 per cent and may contribute to about a third of all traffic accidents. British researchers suggest that sleepiness surpasses alcohol and drugs as the greatest identifiable and preventable cause of accidents in all modes of transport.

Shift work is associated with sleep problems and it seems that industrial accidents are associated with night work, the obvious examples being Chernobyl, Three Mile Island and Bhopal.[4]

LIFESPAN, LIFE QUALITY AND OXIDATION

Medical sleep experts suggest that death appears to occur earlier in patients who get less than five hours of sleep per night.[5] A survey of over one million men and women between 30 — 102 years of age showed that the best survival was among those who slept seven hours per night. Those who slept less than 3.5 — 4.5 hours or more than 8.5 hours experienced higher death rates.[6] The design of this study was criticized; however a survey of a million people is not a trivial study and even if excessively long or short sleep duration does not increase death rates, it does have negative effects on health and wellbeing.

Alcoholics have less delta (slow wave) restorative sleep and more REM sleep, and they are at risk of a number of diseases and infections. Sleep disorders in alcoholics are known to affect the immune system by reducing natural killer cells that protect us from infections.

You may be bombarded about the antioxidant benefits of alcohol but keep in mind that alcohol's adverse effects include addiction, liver and brain damage, breast development in men, weight problems, gastritis, sleep disorders and alcoholic dementia. I consider that a healthy daily level of alcohol is one standard serve for women and two for men.

Relatively high oxidation coupled with the generation of harmful free radicals occurs during the day as a result of your body's normal metabolic activities, as well as from physical activity and exposure to pollutants. While you are resting at night there is less oxidation and, consequently, free radicals are more easily neutralized.[7]

> This is why sleep is said to be the best antioxidant and the best anti-ageing elixir.

DISEASES AND SLEEP

Sleep is likely to be cancer preventive because healthful sleep is linked to higher levels of the sleep hormone melatonin, which has antioxidant effects.

A survey of breast cancer patients indicated that 63 per cent of the women reported one or more types of sleep disturbance and 37 per cent had used sleeping pills.[8] It was found that those whose breast cancer had spread to the bone were more likely to have sleeping problems but in addition they were less educated, more depressed, in pain and lacked social support. As you will see under the next heading, a good night's sleep also encourages an appropriate level of adrenal stress hormones and special immune cells, both of which relate to wellbeing and cancer recovery.

The pineal gland, located within the brain, secretes melatonin, a hormone involved in the sleep-wake cycle and which generally peaks between 1 a.m. to 2 a.m. There is some evidence that melatonin has a protective effect against cancer. Shift workers, such as nurses who are exposed to light at night, have lower melatonin levels, and a large study found that women who work rotating nights shifts, face an increased risk of colon cancer.[9]

IMMUNE FUNCTION, GLUCOSE METABOLISM AND STRESS

Brain cells that are involved in sleep are linked to the immune system. For instance, patients with the flu often say that they sleep for long periods of time — and this might reflect the 'body wisdom.' When fighting an infection, your immune system produces chemicals called cytokines, some of which are sleep inducing. That's why practitioners should prescribe rest as part of infection treatment because rest apparently allows your immune system to do its job better.

Loss of sleep may increase C-reactive protein, an inflammatory marker of cardiovascular risk that is produced in your body.[10] A survey of 71617 nurses indicated that those who had more than nine hours sleep and less than seven hours had a slightly increased risk of heart disease.[11]

Sleep restriction may lead to impaired glucose metabolism and may be a risk factor for developing diabetes.[12] Exercise, regular eating patterns and non-processed foods are recommended for preventing both diabetes and insomnia. Diabetics with sleep problems should consult their doctor because they may have nighttime blood sugar fluctuations.

People suffering from bereavement-related depression spent three nights in a sleep laboratory and were monitored throughout the night. Stress-related intrusive thoughts and avoidance behaviors were linked to greater time awake and this was associated with lower numbers of circulating natural killer cells. A decrease in these particular lymphocyte cells indicates lowered immune function, making the body more vulnerable to infections and diseases.[13] No one is excluded from varying degrees of grief and trauma and accompanying sleepless nights, but this study confirms that you should get help for stress that continually disrupts sleep.

WELLBEING AND HAPPINESS

A poll by the National Sleep Foundation, USA, found that lack of sleep caused impatience and aggravation, as well as *increased appetite*. Sleep debt also has a harmful impact on carbohydrate metabolism and it lowers thyrotropin, a thyroid-stimulating hormone released by the pituitary. These effects may lead to increased bodyweight and low energy. This is why there are media reports advising that adequate sleep helps you lose weight — although excess sleep obviously has the opposite effect.

Studies show that people with long-term sleep disorders between the ages of 14 to 84 years, are prone to depression.[14]

Daytime sleepiness is a measure of insomnia and this includes your likelihood of dozing off while reading, chatting, watching TV, as a car passenger, and/or as a driver while stopping for a few minutes in traffic.[15] Occasionally this may happen to all of us for various reasons, such as boredom or shift work, but a high rate of dozing off during the day indicates a sleep problem — or very old age.

Compared to good sleepers, poor sleepers tend to have faster heart rates, lower ratings for concentration, relaxation, and movement skills, and less favorable brain wave activities.

A sleep debt increases the evening blood levels of the hormone cortisol and hypes up the primitive part of the nervous system.[16] This means that your body is primed for 'fight or flight' rather than rest and repose, even though you may not be feeling energetic. That's why insomniacs often say they feel exhausted but can't sleep.

ECONOMY

Inadequate sleep costs millions of dollars a year in sick days and accidents.

IN CONCLUSION

The above are a few examples of the effects of sleep problems on wellbeing. Some people have the illogical opinion that they should have as little sleep as possible, yet very few consciously choose to have as few nutrients as possible even though sleep is just as important as a healthy diet for wellbeing.

You might consider the cascade effects of various disorders.

A few examples:

- If you are sleep-deprived you handle stress poorly. Do you complain incessantly about the stress in your life? Is your stress really worse than that of others? Do your friends and colleagues want to hear your continual complaints? Is your social life diminishing and are you feeling down? Perhaps the real problem is that sleep deprivation has affected your nervous system to the degree that you can't effectively cope with common daily hassles? This lack of coping may weaken your resistance to infections and then your energy and work suffer as well as your social life.

- You can get by with a little sleep but this may cause inflammation leading to stomach problems that in turn may affect what you eat. The inflammation also means that you will not be absorbing nutrients as effectively and it is thought that about 50 per cent of diseases are caused by insufficient essential nutrients.

A balance of work or study, some routine, learning new things, exercise, socializing, relaxation and sleep, seems the best formula. You simply must organise your life so that you have a variety of experiences, including adequate restorative sleep. This organization may need to include setting priorities so that you don't cram too much into each day and consequently lose your capacity to understand your real needs and the needs of others. Don't wait until you become so exhausted that you can't even sleep!

I hope this chapter has given you evidence that you must organise your life so that you get *your* full sleep requirements rather than limiting your sleeping hours in the mistaken belief that you have more important things to do.

Chapter 3

CAUSES OF INSOMNIA

When you look at the long list of causes in this chapter, you may wonder how any of us manage to get any sleep! Even if a specific disease causes insomnia, it is sensible to do everything possible to reduce the effects of the disease because lack of sleep may make the illness worse, which in turn may cause other problems and worsen the insomnia. Nothing in your body works in isolation.

There's always a cause for insomnia!

The cause may be physical, genetic, nutritional, emotional, mental or behavioral, meaning that you simply prefer other nocturnal activities rather than sleep.

Factors that impede restorative sleep are listed below:

1. Ageing
2. Alcohol - excess
3. Allergies
4. Altitude - high
5. Anxiety
6. Apnoea
7. Arthritis and muscle/joint pain
8. Bad experiences
9. Bedroom environment
10. Biological sleep clock (circadian rhythm) disorders
11. Bladder and kidney problems

12. Bowel and intestinal problems

13. Changes in lifestyle or sleeping environment

14. Chemicals, moulds and odors

15. Cigarette smoking

16. Coffee and caffeine-containing drinks

17. Colors – too stimulating

18. Depression

19. Dietary deficiencies

20. Dietary excesses and irregularities

21. Digestive problems

22. Diseases and disorders

23. Drugs, social — *see also* withdrawal symptoms

24. Eating disorders and fasting

25. Electromagnetic sensitivity

26. Exercise deficiency

27. Exercise excess

28. Fears

29. Fluid intake — excessive or dehydration

30. Genetic influences

31. Heart and circulatory diseases

32. Herbal stimulants and tonics

33. Hormone imbalances

34. Immune dysfunction

35. Itching skin

36. Jet lag

37. Light and dark excesses or insufficiencies

38. Modern lifestyle

39. Mouth breathing (nasal, sinus or respiratory congestion)

40. Neurological diseases

41. Nightmares and disturbing dreams
42. Night sweats
43. Nocturnal myoclonus (muscle contractions)
44. Noise
45. Obesity
46. Overwork
47. Pain and stiffness
48. Pets
49. Pharmaceuticals – prescribed medications
50. Physical discomfort
51. Psychiatric disorders
52. Psychological stress
53. Respiratory infections and diseases
54. Restless leg syndrome
55. Seizures and serious brain disorders or tumors
56. Sex deprivation
57. Shift work
58. Sleeping position
59. Sleep routine insufficiency
60. Snoring
61. Spiritual poverty
62. Temperature, inappropriate
63. Thoughts
64. Tinnitus (often associated with dizziness)
65. Trauma and grief
66. Winding down requirements
67. Withdrawal symptoms
68. Worrying about sleep!

1... AGEING

Sleep becomes somewhat shorter, shallower and fragmented in the elderly although large-scale surveys indicate that about a third of the older population sleep well, so ageing itself should not be considered synonymous with insomnia. Some older people might function more effectively if they have more sleep but pharmaceutical drugs are rarely the best or total solution.

In older people, metabolism slows down about ten per cent and physical activity is reduced by about fifteen per cent. Putting on weight and lack of exercise contribute to many health problems that directly or indirectly impair quality and length of sleep. Obviously, insufficient exercise contributes to joint and circulatory problems that cause pain and discomfort; and obesity may cause pressure on the bladder leading to the urge to urinate during the night.

Lack of restorative sleep in any age group means daytime fatigue and this contributes to a wide range of unhealthy habits, such as sedentary lifestyles and coffee or sugar 'hits' to keep you going. Overcoming the cycle of unhealthy lifestyle and poor sleep is difficult but worthwhile — even for very elderly people. It's disgraceful to imply that there is no point in implementing a health program for the elderly — and dispiriting for the individual. A number of my elderly patients are hurt and angry because practitioners indicate in various ways that certain treatments are not an option because they are too expensive, too long-term and so on.

2... ALCOHOL, EXCESS

Although alcohol appears to be relaxing and it generally promotes the onset of sleep, it reduces the total sleep time. A survey of young adults found that those who reported needing only six hours of sleep had a higher alcoholic intake and had started drinking at an earlier age compared with those who required more sleep.

Some insomniacs choose alcohol because they believe it will numb their anxieties but actually alcohol excess leads to diminished sleep and rebound anxiety.

Some effects of alcohol are given below:

- Alcohol reduces the amount of REM sleep in the first half of sleep, and in the later part of sleep it increases REM sleep and increases light sleep.[1] In other words, it changes the timing of the different types of sleep thereby affecting the way that your brain processes information, as well as reducing the level of deep restorative sleep.

- It interferes with the normal actions of brain chemicals (neurotransmitters) such as gamma-aminobutyric acid (GABA) and glutamate. For instance, GABA has some necessary inhibitory effects while glutamate is excitatory and involved with wakefulness.[2] In other words, alcohol interferes with the brain's function of counterbalancing activity and repose.

- Even after alcohol is no longer detected in the blood, reaction time and alertness, remain diminished. In a study of young pilots who drank sufficient quantities to result in blood alcohol levels of 0.10 and 0.12 per cent, performance in a flight simulator was impaired more than fourteen hours after consuming the alcohol, compared to performance after consuming a placebo.[3]

- Alcohol reduces growth hormone. Growth hormone is involved in producing new cells and has other important functions, as outlined in this chapter under the heading 'hormone imbalances'.

Alcohol is complicated because it has both stimulating and sedative effects, but long-term alcohol excess actually causes depression and irrationality rather than happiness and congeniality — as anyone who has lived with a heavy drinker knows.

Some people find that even a few drinks will make them sleepy but they wake in the middle of the night and then can't get back to sleep. Having a 'nightcap' is no longer recommended because people rapidly develop tolerance to alcohol, which means that after a relatively short period of time, you need more than a single nightcap to satisfy you.

35

A safe daily alcohol intake is probably one serve for women and two for men — although sensitive people may not tolerate even this modest intake, particularly late at night. Insomniacs should not drink alcohol after dinner and I suggest having one alcohol-free day each week.

3... ALLERGIES

Anything that irritates your body is likely to prevent or reduce sleep. Inhaled allergens will cause nasal blockages or asthmatic symptoms; external allergens will make your skin itchy; and food allergies and sensitivities may cause digestive upsets, abdominal pain or diarrhoea. As far as practicable find and eliminate allergens or get treatment to at least reduce their adverse effects. If symptoms persist get a referral to an allergy specialist for testing and perhaps an elimination diet. If you are found to be allergic to dust mites, pull up the bed room carpet and have nice clean tiles or polished floor boards on the bedroom floor.

4... ALTITUDE

If lowlanders move to altitudes above 3200 metres their sleep may be markedly disturbed for a week or more. At relatively higher altitudes, reduced oxygen levels make breathing less effective, and therefore the heart has to pump faster. During a skiing or trekking holiday you may not sleep well (in spite of the outdoor exercise) and you may be conscious of your heartbeat, particularly if you're lying awake at night longing for sleep. At altitudes above 4000—5000 metres adaptation may be quite prolonged and uncomfortable without oxygen enrichment, and the circadian rhythm may be disrupted. Taking ginkgo herb and a vitamin E or antioxidant supplement may help the body adjust to high altitude changes.

5... ANXIETY

Anxiety is a common cause of insomnia. Severe anxiety requires practitioner help otherwise it disrupts everyday activities and relationships.

If worries and unwanted thoughts come at night instead of sleep, tell yourself that you will think about these things tomorrow at a certain time. Sometimes people allocate a 'daily worry time', others write down their emotional problems, put the list in a drawer and therefore out of sight during the evening. Continuously and ineffectively trying to solve a problem can sometimes make it worse — as you will see under the heading 'thoughts' in this chapter.

You may become habituated to certain actions even though they are not successful, and you may need someone to point you in another direction. For instance, patients often say they have been on a particular treatment or remedy for months, or years, but their health problem has not improved. Some can't even say why they started a particular treatment or remedy.

If you are told to sit or lie quietly and 'watch your thoughts'; you may find that when you *try* this exercise that your mind seems empty. Telling people not to worry, but to relax and be absolutely still, may send their minds into a whirl of activity and produce urges to think, move and twitch. Of course, reactions are variable. Some adults relax when they listen to a distracting story; others relax at the sounds of a mantra being chanted, while others respond to standard relaxation therapy or stretching exercises.

If I'm angry or upset about something, rather than going to bed and having the same irritating thoughts go round and round in my brain, I write a frank letter to whoever I believe is responsible, and this often expels much of the emotion. Then I tell myself I've done all I can for the day. Next day, I read it through, and destroy it — or tone it down, make it constructive criticism and send it; so that I feel I have taken some action rather than bottling up the irritation. *Never* send critical notes or letters to friends and family, as you should discuss your feelings verbally — and do this when you feel calm. None of us is perfect and usually it's better to let incidents 'wash over you' rather than discuss them and run the risk of an argument. You need other people, you don't need to have the last word, the world is definitely not short of people who criticise, and praise generates happiness.

If you put a handful of salt into a small bowl it will be too salty to drink. If you put the same quantity into a river, the river does not suffer and everyone will be able to drink the water. In the same way, if your heart is small, one unjust word will cause you suffering.
Buddha -
(This advice was offered over 2000 years ago before our rivers were polluted)

Diverting your thoughts when you are trying to sleep may work better than trying to erase them or counting sheep. One suggestion is to have a non-stimulating mental exercise. For instance, imagine that you have a country retreat and picture the house and the land, and how you might redecorate the interior and the garden to make it your own sanctuary for peace and healing. Or you might take an imaginary trip to your favorite place and aim to visualize every detail. Another option is to read, or listen to an audio disk or cassette as discussed under 'sleep routine insufficiency' in this chapter — or do the exercises given in Appendix II and III.

Believing that you *must* have a specified number of hours of sleep; or having your own thoughts delude you that sleep is elusive and unpredictable, may cause more anxiety and reinforce your insomnia. You can be your own therapist by using some of the techniques in this book. If your own efforts aren't successful, I suggest you find a hypnotherapist or a psychologist. It may take between two to eight sessions to modify your beliefs and thought patterns. Being a 'worrier' and poor sleeper may be part of your genes, your personality or your habits, so you may need an occasional follow up treatment.

6... APNOEA

Apnoea is a combination of suspended breathing and snoring during sleep. Repeated pauses in breathing result in less oxygen being carried throughout the body, which in turn may lead to headaches, fatigue, mood swings, memory loss, inability to concentrate and loss of libido. Every cell in your body needs a steady supply of oxygen and you should get medical advice for sleep apnoea because it is linked to a higher incidence of heart problems, high blood pressure, stroke and accidents.

Severe sleep apnoea has very dangerous consequences; a study in The Lancet journal showed that severe sleep apnoea increases the risk of fatal cardiovascular disease even more than smoking or high blood pressure does.

Snoring may be drying or irritating to the mouth, throat and lungs. Loud snoring followed by periodic silence is distressing to bed partners.

Sleep apnoea is linked to lower levels of female sex hormones.[4] Decreased testosterone levels are also linked to obstructive sleep apnea.[5] Testosterone increases sex-drive and energy, and correcting nighttime breathing patterns might increase libido. Other hormonal disturbances related to sleep apnoea include imbalances in growth hormone and thyroid hormone.

MRI scan research indicates that people with sleep apnoea may have some damage to the part of the brain that controls speech and almost 40 per cent of patients scanned had a history of childhood speech impediments such as stammering.

Obesity, alcohol, sleeping pills, sedatives and sleeping on the back may worsen apnoea. However, apnoea treatment is not as simple as correcting lifestyle shortcomings or taking a herbal remedy.

Central Sleep Apnoea

In this category of apnoea, there is no throat obstruction but repeated interruptions of breathing cause sleep disruptions and daytime fatigue. The brain is not properly monitoring oxygen and carbon dioxide levels during sleep. Snoring does *not* usually occur in this type of apnoea.

Obstructive Sleep Apnoea

In this form of apnoea part of the throat tissue closes off the airway to the lungs and this occurs in about two per cent of women and up to six per cent of men. The brain wakes the sleeping person in order to activate the muscle tone in the throat, and this awakening can occur many times during the night.

Sometimes the mouth, throat, tongue or jaws are shaped in such a way that apnoea is more likely to occur. The bones and tissues in the face and throat are specifically different in those suffering from obstructive sleep apnea.[6]

Upper Airway Resistance Syndrome

This is a condition where the patient does not stop breathing but the body has to work extra hard to supply adequate oxygen. The usual outcome is lighter sleep coupled with daytime fatigue. Whatever the breathing impairment, it is obviously sensible to do all you can to get a good intake of oxygen because it is not only essential for life but also for wellbeing.

Habitual breathing through your mouth may indirectly lead to sleep apnoea and daytime fatigue. You should breathe in through your nose because this filters the air and ensures that the air is the right temperature when it reaches the lungs. Constant mouth breathing will dry the mouth and throat, and may cause gagging, coughing or upset the lungs; and may wake you because of the discomfort. If your nose is severely blocked get practitioner advice about treatment. I have given a few simple treatments for clearing nasal passages in Chapter 5 and also on page 89.

The treatment of sleep apnoea depends on the severity of the problem. In mild cases, treatment may include reducing alcohol intake and having absolutely no alcohol after dinner, or a weight loss program or a tennis ball may be sown into the back of the pyjamas to discourage back sleeping.

There are different types of sleep apnoea and a definite diagnosis is made by an overnight study in a sleep laboratory with electrodes being taped to various parts of the body and scalp to monitor breathing and sleep quality. What seems to be just a case of irritating snoring may indeed be a complex health problem, so we need to be understanding about snorers and encourage them to get proper medical diagnosis and treatment for their health.

Specific Devices To Treat Sleep Apnoea

Medical and dental options include various types of masks, jaw supports or devices worn in the mouth. Most people find these somewhat uncomfortable at the beginning but generally they soon find that the benefits make it worthwhile. There are devices that can be medically prescribed and a nasal continuous positive airway pressure (nCPAP) device has been tested for moderate to severe apnoea and shown to be substantially helpful.[7] Indeed apart from giving you a good night's sleep, nCPAP treatment can be life saving, and reduce the increased risk of cardiovascular deaths back to normal based on the results of a 10-year follow up study of 1400 men with sleep apnoea.

Surgery may be appropriate in some cases.

Snoring is covered later in this chapter. There are various over over-the-counter anti-snoring devices available in pharmacies and some health food stores but these do not correct apnoea.

Caution: If apnoea is suspected, do not use medications that reduce breathing, such as sedatives and sleeping pills. Apnoea should be treated because this not only improves quality of life for patients but also for their bed partners and families. It is stressful enough being kept awake by someone snoring but even worse if you are anxiously listening to check that the breathing is going to restart.

7... ARTHRITIS AND JOINT/MUSCLE PAIN

Pain and discomfort obviously reduce sleep. Remedies that may help degenerative and inflammatory arthritis include:

• Glucosamine, chondroitin sulphate and MSM.

• Lyprinol, ginger, turmeric, gota kola and many other herbs.

• Dietary changes such as increasing raw vegetables and fruits, raw vegetable juicing and raw nuts and seeds and oily fish

• Fish oil and flaxseed oil capsules

• Bone and Joint Nutrient capsules containing a combination of glucosamine with other minerals (calcium hydroxyapatite, boron, manganese, silica, zinc, magnesium, copper) and vitamin D. For more information call the Health Advisory line on 0246 558855

• A varied exercise program that is appropriate to age and joint condition.

When 150 American children and adults with persistent muscle and bone pain were examined, it was found that 93 per cent of them were deficient in vitamin D.[8] Few foods contain vitamin D so we should get the bulk of this vitamin from the sun, via the skin. In Australia this vitamin should not be lacking, however, sunblocks reduce the capacity of the skin to produce vitamin D by 95 per cent and many people do not get sunlight on their skin because of ethnic beliefs or because they are worried about skin cancer. Vitamin D is needed for bones and muscles; for organ function, immune modulation, insulin secretion and it may prevent hypertension, heart disease and some cancers. My suggestion is that everyone should get outdoor exercise with at least our arms and legs exposed for 30 minutes daily, preferably at sunrise or before 9 a.m. Eat vitamin D rich foods such as egg yolks and oily fish and in the winter take a cod liver oil capsule daily. If you have persistent aches and pains that interfere with sleep ask your doctor to do a blood test to measure your levels of vitamin D – you may get a shock! Pain is depressing. Sometimes it is necessary to take painkillers or non-steroidal anti-inflammatory drugs, and some natural therapies may help you reduce the quantity of pharmaceuticals that you need. If you don't treat joint and muscle pain the result may be insomnia, a sedentary lifestyle and reduced quality of life.

8... BAD EXPERIENCES

Getting attacked in bed, or elsewhere, is a nasty experience that stays with you forever. It serves no purpose telling people not to worry or to get on with their lives. You only have to hear the daily news to know that we all need to be reasonably cautious. You can have counselling and tell yourself that you're not going to let some maniac ruin your life but the incident is strongly embedded in your brain. However, if you've been attacked while sleeping you'd have to be extremely unlucky to have a repeat experience.

Some people find the night particularly scary because of frightening experiences or fears, and compensate by having a light on all night in the bedroom, but as you will see later in this chapter, light is an impediment to sleep. Others have a security lock fitted on the inside of the bedroom door, or even have a metal grill put on the outside of the door and then become anxious in case there is a fire or an emergency. One trick is to sleep with the door key attached on a neck lace so you can find it in an instant and keep your fully-charged mobile phone by the bed side. It's reassuring to be prepared.

I suggest that you keep the bedroom dark and if you are worried about someone entering the room while you are asleep, put a large, heavily framed picture (or something similar) against the inside of the door at a slight angle, and then there will be a loud crash if someone begins to open the door from the outside. If you have carpet, you could place a flat piece of metal for the picture to fall on. You can also buy hand-held alarms or get special alarms fitted in appropriate areas inside the house. It will help allay your fears, if you have adequate overall security for your house including some lights (not in the bedroom) that turn on and off periodically during the night — and a big dog or a big, brave partner. In addition, do a self-defence course; it's good exercise and gives you more confidence. Trust in God, consider the unlikely probability of harm to yourself, but *always* regularly review your home security and physical strength.

9... BEDROOM ENVIRONMENT

Poor sleepers should take a look at their bedroom furniture because even relatively mild discomfort will wake some people. Insomniacs have the unfortunate tendency to look for any little thing that might prevent or disrupt their sleep – even a wrinkled sheet may be annoying!

You spend more time in bed than you do in your car so it is important to consider quality when choosing the right bed and setting for you. During the 1980's, researchers in the USA found that a rocking bed reduced night time waking in people with respiratory weakness. Although rocking beds are not available in Australia you can buy waterbeds or vibration mattresses that may improve your sleep. Tilt beds can be of great assistance in those with reflux (heartburn) or respiratory conditions, though most people sleep most efficiently when laying down, horizontally.

Our budgets will often determine the type of bedding we buy, though when choosing a mattress you should test it against your own body weight. 'Economy' mattresses are closely packed with filling and may retain moisture, which will affect your body temperature and breathing. Firmer is not necessarily better especially if you have back problems.[9] Whichever mattress you choose it can take a few days or even weeks to settle into a new mattress. It is often considered that a fully sprung spring base is more supportive and comfortable than a wooden base.

A woollen underlay may provide a cost effective method to improve your sleep.[10] Wool is nature's miracle fibre. It has a complex structure which gives it unique qualities, ideal for bedding. Wool is water repellent but moisture absorbent and this unusual combination helps the body's natural cooling process by encouraging moisture to evaporate away from the skin, so that you maintain an even temperature as you sleep. Wool can absorb up to 30% of its own weight in moisture, without feeling damp. Because of its natural crimp and loft, wool also acts as a great insulator, keeping you warm in cold conditions. Independent research shows that when sleeping on, under and with wool, you have a lower, more consistent heart rate, sleep more peacefully and wake more refreshed. Wool is also naturally non-allergenic, flame resistant and environmentally friendly, making it safer for the whole family.

Restless sleepers may find that a 100 per cent down pillow is the best choice because it gently supports the neck and will change shape if you move. Consider any allergies or sensitivity you may have to the pillow filling, and if in doubt, choose a non-allergenic make of pillow. You need to shop around and choose a pillow firmness that suits your body shape, weight and sleeping patterns. Larger, heavier people often find a firmer pillow more comfortable and supportive for their neck. Pillows will lose their integrity and should be updated every few years. Check with the retailer for the manufacturer's warranty and instructions. The same considerations should also be made to your bed linen. Cotton is preferred to synthetic fibres, and will be more conducive to natural sleeping patterns, and is less likely to cause irritation and excess sweating.

10... BIOLOGICAL SLEEP CLOCK DISORDERS

Although the control centre of our biological sleep clock is in the brain, there is speculation that we also have minor clocks in other parts of the body and these receive and presumably modify information from the primary clock, and also operate independently. Some people may have a primary biological sleep clock that is somewhat different from 24 hours, and it may be quite difficult to re-set.

When we change our environment and lifestyle, the sleep

clock attempts to re-set itself in order to help our wellbeing. Researchers in the high arctic were monitored during a period of constant daylight and the majority of them developed a sleep-wake cycle longer than 24 hours.[11]

Circadian sleep disorders are generally divided into two categories: Early sleepiness/early awakening; and late sleepiness/ late awakening. In my clinic, the most common disorder is late bedtime and desired late awakening. Some of my fatigued patients tell me that they simply like being up late although a few say they don't like going to bed. The night may be their enjoyment or relaxation time, when they feel free to do what they want — or 'me time'. There is a lot of interesting entertainment and things to do at night compared to what people had sixty years ago, when they used to sit around chatting, gazing into the fire, knitting or playing cards. However, the problem is that indulgence in nighttime entertainment doesn't combine with having to get up early to go to work or get children off to school. This evening indulgence needs to be restricted unless you can get up late the next day, because long-term sleep deprivation can lead to health and social problems. If you're in this category I suggest you follow the recommendations below under 'sleep routine insufficiency'. The first retraining strategy is to get up somewhat earlier than customary and to get outside in the early morning light. You might also make your bedroom more pleasurable. Indulge in a sheepskin mattress overlay, a lavender pillow, some relaxing music or perhaps audio books.

For those who go to bed very early and consequently wake very early, this may not seem a problem and you may enjoy spending an hour or so by yourself in the morning. However, your sleep pattern may be out of sync with your family and friends and may limit your social life. You could try having exposure to very bright lights in the evening for about two hours. The idea of the evening light is to trick your biological clock into thinking it is still activity time. Start going to bed 15 minutes later and over a period of months you could try further extending bedtime. Changing decades of sleep habits is a gradual and often a difficult process.

Although your biological sleep clock can tolerate some deviations, it functions better if regular bedtimes and wake times are maintained, even on weekends and holidays. *Remember that the ideal time for sleep is between 10 p.m. to 6 a.m. because this seems to improve brain function.*

In the USA and Europe, various types of light therapy units are available for treating circadian rhythm disorders, and jet lag. These units are sometimes referred to as 'light boxes' and contain full-spectrum or cool-white fluorescent tubes with about 2500-lux illumination, which is five times the level of typical indoor lighting. Depending on the disorder and severity, the patient sits or works close to the light for specified times, but it is not necessary to stare into the light. The Australian experts to whom I spoke were not in favour of light boxes. I don't think they are necessary because the *outdoor* light is remarkably strong in Australia, even on overcast days. More information is given in this chapter under 'light and dark excesses or insufficiencies'.

11... BLADDER AND KIDNEY PROBLEMS

When you sleep, your kidneys automatically function so that urine becomes more concentrated and less fluid goes to the bladder. As we age, this kidney function becomes less efficient and many older people are woken to urinate during the night. If you are woken more than once, I suggest you see a practitioner or physiotherapist to learn pelvic floor exercises which will often help greatly.

Nocturia (nighttime urination) has many causes including excess fluid intake, cardiovascular problems, urine infections, diabetes, menopause, constipation, obesity, pregnancy, prolapse of the bladder, dysfunction of the nerves to the bladder, and kidney diseases etc. Alcohol and diuretic drugs are other causes of nocturia.

Basically, anything that causes irritation or pressure on the bladder produces the urge to urinate. In men prostate gland enlargement (Benign Prostatic Hypertrophy or BPH) is a common cause of urinary frequency and may be associated with a weak urinary flow and delayed onset of urination.

If your sleep is being disturbed by frequent and/or excess urination please see your doctor for a urine test. If the problem persists see a specialist urologist, as there will be a treatable cause. Infections and diabetes are easily treated so that the urinary frequency goes away. If you have a chronic or recurrent infection in the urine that becomes resistant to antibiotics, you will need to use nutritional medicine to overcome the problem. I recommend that you start to juice regularly using things such as celery, radish, carrot, ginger root, capsicum, cucumber, apple, cranberry and red onion. You can also add a dash of raw garlic to the juice, as garlic is a powerful antibiotic. Add a half teaspoon of "MSM Plus vitamin C powder" to your juice and you will further cleanse the urine and reduce bacterial contamination of the urine. Taking a regular supplement of vitamin C and the mineral selenium can prevent or reduce urinary tract infections.

Menopausal women may have thinning and weakening (atrophy) of the tissues of the vagina and bladder leading to nocturnal urinary frequency and burning. This can be easily overcome with a cream containing natural oestrogen, which is applied twice weekly to the outside of the vagina (the vulva). You will need a doctor's script for this hormonal cream.

In some patients there is a hyperactivity or over activity of the nerves to the bladder and this causes the need to pass small amounts of urine repetitively during the night; obviously this is very annoying as it serves no purpose. It may be associated with a sense of urgency to pass urine, as the bladder is not well controlled. In such cases a very small dose of a pharmaceutical drug called a tricyclic drug can calm the bladder nerves down to normal. Examples of such drugs are Doxepin or Tryptanol and often only a small dose of say 10mg is needed and this is best taken at 7 p.m. each night. These small doses of tricyclic drugs do not usually have any side effects and may finally enable you to get that sleep destroying bladder of yours under control.

In men with prostate gland enlargement natural remedies such as the herbs saw palmetto, nettle root, epilobium and red clover and the mineral selenium can help to reduce symptoms. These men will find that certain dietary changes can help to shrink the enlarged prostate gland and these include – eating more legumes (beans, lentils and peas), sprouts, ground flaxseeds and more vegetables.

As far as practicable and safe, do not put on bright lights if you wake during the night to visit the bathroom, because the light may stop your brain's production of the sleep hormone melatonin. Alternatively, use a small torch or have a very dim hall light. Never rush to the bathroom at night especially in dim light as it is easy to fall over when you are groggy.

12... BOWEL AND INTESTINAL PROBLEMS

Anything that causes pain is likely to wake you. Colic, bloating and inflammatory intestinal diseases are obvious examples.

Severe constipation may cause discomfort and put pressure on the bladder and then you will get the urge to urinate. Look into your diet as you are probably lacking fibre and may also not be drinking enough fluids during the day. Strategies to increase fibre are usually effective and include grinding (in a coffee grinder or food processor) a combination of equal amounts of flaxseeds, almonds and sunflower seeds and eating 1 to 2 tablespoons daily. Keep this mixture in the freezer. The product called Fibretone is an excellent source of natural fibre.

Avoid eating large meals late at night; if you are late for dinner, have a small light low-fat meal. Those with nocturnal indigestion can usually benefit from strong digestive enzymes taken with the evening meal such as pancrease capsules. If the problem persists see a specialist gastroenterologist.

13... CHANGES IN LIFESTYLE OR ENVIRONMENT

When your environment changes, aim to follow your usual routine are far as practicable and take a few familiar bedroom items with you, such as your own pillow, your favorite disks, a photo, your 'lavender teddy bear' and so on. When I'm away from home I always take a book with me and aim to stay up somewhat later than usual.

Some of my patients complain that they have problems adjusting to daylight saving because changing the time one hour upsets their biological rhythm and causes fatigue for days — or even weeks.

14... CHEMICALS, MOULDS AND ODORS

An American doctor suggests that fire retardant chemicals in mattresses may contribute to SIDS (sudden infant death syndrome) because fungi and other microorganisms consume chemicals (phosphorus, arsenic and antimony) in the fire retardant plastic polyvinyl chloride mattress pad. The microorganisms emit neurotoxic gases (phosphine, arsine and stibine) and when the human warms the mattress body these odorless gases rise up and are inhaled. Apparently the nervous system is damaged if this continues long-term, and the solution is to use a mattress pad that is not made from polyvinyl chloride.[12]

I could not find any evidence that there is a problem in adults but many chemicals, including some common pesticides, are known to disrupt the nervous system and if you have insomnia that doesn't respond to other treatments this is another factor for you to consider.

It is also possible that your mattress contains mould or fungi and it may help to air the mattress in the sun periodically. You can also add 6 to 10 drops of tea tree oil to the washing machine, as it helps to kill all types of micro-organisms in bed linen.

It seems that pleasant smells are relaxing and engender positive thoughts, so it is possible that unpleasant smells could cause agitation and negative thinking, and consequently disrupt sleep. Aromatherapy is covered in Chapter 5.

15... CIGARETTE SMOKING

Heavy smokers tend to sleep lightly and have less REM sleep. They may wake up after about four hours of sleep because they have nicotine withdrawal. Cigarette smoking is also known to interfere with blood flow and lung function, both of which can cause problems that are linked to poor sleep, such as cramps and oxygen deficit.

16... COFFEE AND CAFFEINE-CONTAINING DRINKS

Insomniacs may need to completely eliminate caffeine-containing drinks, including cola, because tests indicate that caffeine takes longer to be eliminated from the bodies of poor sleepers. Others may tolerate a few 'caffeine' drinks in the early part of the day. (Good sleepers often have a cup of coffee before bed!) Common tea and coffee both contain theophylline as well as caffeine, and both these compounds have stimulatory effects. Common tea is far less stimulatory than coffee.

Black and green tea contain powerful antioxidants and these teas are generally recommended. Even if tea is *not* stimulatory for you, don't have too much fluid after dinner because there's a limit to the capacity of the human bladder.

17... COLORS

Relaxing colors include green, blue, mauve, and purple. I suggest avoiding bright colors and bright lights in the bedroom even though I doubt that you actually detect or 'feel' colors once you put the lights out! However, it is possible that bright colors stimulate you before you turn off the light.

18... DEPRESSION

There are varying degrees and types of depression and generally depression is accompanied by slow wave sleep abnormalities and waking during the night. In some cases insomnia causes depression and in other cases clinical depression causes insomnia.

In cold climates where the days are short, some people get winter depression (Seasonal Affective Disorder or SAD). They are constantly fatigued, and may also sleep excessively and crave sugars. In Europe and North America, light therapy helps this condition but in Australia all you need to do is get outside — especially in the early morning light.

For both depression and insomnia you may wish to start with natural treatments and remedies, as these can often work very effectively. They do not provide a "quick fix" and may take 2 to 3 months to really help the depression.

Natural Therapies For Depression Include –

1. The herb St John's wort can help mild cases of depression and insomnia. I have found that this herb works better if it is taken in a tablet that combines it with B group vitamins and minerals. For more information call the Health Advisory Service on 0246 558855.

2. Supplements of omega 3 fatty acids. The brain is largely composed of fat, but not just any old fat! Two thirds of the weight of the brain is composed of omega 3 polyunsaturated fatty acids and guess what? Your body is unable to manufacture its own supply of omega 3 fatty acids. The best dietary sources are oily fish and flaxseed oil and breast milk, but that can be hard to come by! If your brain is not working efficiently – in other words you cannot sleep, your memory is foggy and your mood is down - it may be due to a deficiency of omega 3 fatty acids and thankfully this is easy to correct.

The best dietary sources of brain boosting omega 3 fatty acids are-

Flaxseed (linseed), hemp-seed oil, pumpkin seeds, walnuts, salmon, sardines, tuna, anchovies, herring, mackerel, marine algae and omega 3 eggs or eggs from free range chickens that are fed flaxseeds, fishmeal and green leafy vegetables.

3. Phospholipids are fats that are found in high amounts in the brain for very good reasons – they form the insulation sheaths around your nerves which keep the electrical circuits running smoothly. There are 2 kinds of phospholipids – phosphatidyl serine and phosphatidyl choline. Good dietary sources include egg yolks and lecithin and I highly recommend these sources for patients with depression, insomnia, poor memory and anxiety.

4. Vitamin C which improves circulation to the brain and reduces brain inflammation.

5. Magnesium tablets can help to re-balance the nervous system and I call magnesium the "great relaxer." You may need 2 to 4 tablets of magnesium complete daily to get good results.

6. Raw juicing using foods such as cabbage, carrot, citrus, ginger root, spinach, beetroot and other green leafy vegetables – this will increase folic acid, which lowers the blood level of the brain-toxic amino acid homocysteine

7. SAMe which can also improve mental energy, although it is quite expensive and is not essential, particularly as you can get your body to make more of its own SAMe if you improve your diet.

19... DIETARY DEFICIENCIES

There are 45 essential nutrients that humans must consume because these nutrients cannot be made in the body from other compounds, and they are required for the body's physical and mental functioning.

In time all strict vegans will become vitamin B12 deficient unless they take a supplement. Elderly people are often short of vitamin B12 either because they don't get enough in the diet or cannot absorb it (pernicious anaemia). They will benefit most from regular 6 weekly injections of vitamin B 12. Vitamin B12 is necessary for the nervous system and a deficiency causes many problems including weakness of the legs, depression, fatigue and insomnia.

The health of your brain and nervous system depends upon adequate amounts of the following fats –

Saturated and mono-unstarurated fat

Omega 3 polyunsaturated fat – especially EPA & DHA

Omega 6 polyunsaturated fat – especially GLA & AA

Cholesterol — cholesterol is found in vast amounts in the healthy human brain and supports your brain's physical and functional integrity.

Make sure that you feed your brain with the fats it needs to function; otherwise it will start to shrink and literally go haywire.

To ensure an adequate dietary intake of healthy brain fats include-

Oily fish (canned fish is fine), a wide variety of raw nuts and seeds, lecithin granules on your cereal, all types of seafood (including crustaceans), whole eggs from free range chickens or omega 3 eggs, cold pressed flaxseed and olive oil, as well as plenty of green leafy vegetables.

In our "fat-phobic" world where people follow low-fat diets in the mistaken belief that they are slimming and healthy, and where doctors are brain washed into believing that their patients should have very low cholesterol levels, we now have a huge number of people who are deficient in the fats essential for healthy brain function. No wonder there is an increasing problem with insomnia and depression. If you are on cholesterol-lowering drugs and feel depressed or cannot sleep, this could be due to the fact that your brain is starved of the cholesterol it needs to function. For the latest information on high cholesterol and the dangers of cholesterol lowering drugs, see the book *Cholesterol the Real Truth* by Dr. Sandra Cabot and Margaret Jasinska ND.

I have found that the most common nutritional deficiencies in those with depression and/or insomnia are –

Fats - omega 3 fatty acids and phospholipids

Vitamin C

Minerals - magnesium and selenium

Further details about nutrients and sleep are given in Chapter 5.

The best way of getting all the essential nutrients is to eat a wide range of foods in as natural a state as possible, and as fresh as possible.

20... DIETARY EXCESSES AND IRREGULARITIES

Bedtime snacks are not generally recommended for insomniacs because food tends to be somewhat warming and stimulating. However, if you have an early dinner and feel hungry at bedtime, or if you have a low blood sugar problem (hypoglycemia), I have given some bedtime snack suggestions in Chapter 5.

It makes sense not to have a large meal before bed but this advice is not always practical if you finish work late and are very hungry by the time you get home at 9 p.m. One way of avoiding an excessively large, late meal is to organise time to have a snack about 3 — 4 p.m. An afternoon snack of vegetable soup, or about one dessertspoon of whey protein in a small tub of plain acidophilus yoghurt or a few nuts and a piece of fruit, provides energy and should reduce the quantity of food you eat late at night.

If you have a large meal just before bed this will increase body temperature and wakefulness, and probably cause abdominal discomfort, and put pressure on your bowel and bladder, all which may prevent sleep or subsequently wake you.

Foods that may be stimulating for insomniacs and best avoided after midday are wheat, corn, sugar and chocolate. In some people the gluten in wheat and other grains may be irritating to the brain; corn is not favorable for blood sugar control and cocoa contains the stimulant theobromine. Having a hot chocolate drink before bed may worsen insomnia.

At all times, choose complex carbohydrates and avoid processed foods especially those with additives, coloring and preservatives because these can irritate the nervous system. Sugar substitutes such as aspartame (Nutrasweet) and sucralose (Splenda) may also be irritating to the brain. Sugars and sugary foods may also cause excess blood glucose levels in some people but sugar in its natural context takes longer to get into the blood and cells compared to refined sugars. Your brain needs glucose while you are sleeping and it's preferable to have this in slow release form from whole foods or from your body stores.

The very worst fats you can eat for your brain's health are called trans fatty acids. After ingested these damaged and mis-shapened fats can be incorporated into your brain to replace the healthy fats like DHA in brain cells. These trans fats are not the right shape for the membranes on your brain cells, so they cause the brain cells to malfunction. Thus you start to find your mental function and perhaps your sleep deteriorating.

Avoid foods with hydrogenated fats containing trans fatty acids by avoiding deep fried foods, hydrogenated vegetable oils (many cheap cooking oils), many margarines, many packaged types of processed foods, chips and donuts. Of course the occasional treat with these junk foods is fine, but if you eat them everyday they will definitely affect your brain function. The only way to avoid these hydrogenated oils and trans fatty acids is to check the labels of the foods you buy – if it appears on the label avoid it as a regular food.

21... DIGESTIVE PROBLEMS

Problems such as ulcers and heartburn (reflux) will cause upper abdominal and/or central chest pain and impede sleep. A common cause of dyspepsia (upper abdominal indigestion) is irregular eating habits or eating too much refined carbohydrate and sugary food. The excess sugar will feed unhealthy bacteria in your stomach leading to imbalances in acid production. An enlarged fatty liver can also press on the stomach causing reflux so it's important to check your liver with an ultrasound scan.

Having *small* regular meals will put less pressure on your digestive system and may help reduce excess stomach acid. Digestive enzymes such as pancrease can be taken with meals to reduce symptoms.

If you have reflux or dyspepsia you should not eat late at night and a light, early dinner is recommended. I suggest practitioner help because your oesophagus and throat are not designed to cope with acid coming up from the stomach, and you need to get a diagnosis as well as a treatment plan. If untreated, the stomach acid can reflux up into the oesophagus and can get inhaled into the larynx and lungs causing a nocturnal cough and a sore throat in the mornings. Natural antacids containing magnesium carbonate and calcium carbonate, aloe vera and the herbs meadowsweet and slippery elm may help a lot. Avoid aluminium containing antacids. In severe cases unless weight is lost, pharmaceutical drugs that reduce stomach acid production can be very effective.

Surveys indicate that reflux problems are sometimes linked to obstructive sleep apnoea and other respiratory problems, including asthma, and reflux is not a problem to be ignored or taken lightly.

22... DISEASES AND DISORDERS

Various diseases including anaemia, cancer, heart, lung and thyroid diseases are linked to poor sleep. Insomnia may be related to either the disease itself or anxiety about the disease. You might think that people with chronic fatigue syndrome sleep excessively but in some cases these patients are exhausted but do not sleep well.

There's always something you can do to improve your health and an option is to consult a health practitioner who is interested in wellbeing as well as disease treatment. You can be seriously ill through no fault of your own and you may need to develop a different philosophy. I have patients who say things like, 'Apart

from the cancer, diabetes and Parkinson's I'm quite healthy'!
You need to find the line between looking after yourself and not
letting your illness take over.

23... DRUGS, SOCIAL —
SEE ALSO WITHDRAWAL SYMPTOMS

Alcohol and coffee have been covered separately in this chapter
and in the context of insomnia they should be considered 'drugs'.
Modest intakes are not harmful for good sleepers but if you stop
taking them for a few days this often shows how addictive they
are because you will probably experience withdrawal headaches,
irritability and perhaps insomnia. Withdrawal symptoms may last
for days or weeks.

Cocaine can seriously disrupt sleep; it changes mood and blood
pressure and increases daytime sleepiness.[13]

Ecstasy (MDMA), speed and various amphetamine-type drugs can
be quite neurotoxic to the serotonergic (wellbeing) system of the
brain.[14]

The immediate effect of speed is obviously increased energy and
endurance, but the long-term effects of stimulants include sleep
disorders.

Stimulant drugs, especially in conjunction with physical activity,
may cause brain hyperthermia (excess heat) which in turn
damages brain cells. Side effects of ecstasy include mental
confusion, exaggerated physical movements and 'midweek
blues', as well as the more serious side effects of serotonin
syndrome which is explained in Appendix IV under antidepressant
medications.

Social drugs impair sleep in specific ways. Ecstasy decreases total
sleep, sleep efficiency, delta (slow wave) sleep and REM sleep.
Cannabis tends to make people groggy and disrupts behavior
and movements. Withdrawal effects of both these drugs include
insomnia.

24... EATING DISORDERS

Eating disorders such as anorexia and bulimia are psychiatric problems that require professional help. These conditions are linked to a range of emotional and physical problems, including sleep disorders.

Rat studies indicate that food restriction reduces the sleep hormone melatonin. You may have read that food restriction prolongs life but this relates to rat studies with their food intake restricted by one-third to one-half. If this level of restriction were applied to a typical human diet, it would result in deficiency diseases. Although the food-restricted rats were more active, they had high levels of stress hormones, and probably slept less. The trouble with many studies is that the public is fed bits of information and the reality is that rats don't complain about insomnia, and semi-starvation is not good for mental and physical wellbeing. Rats are nothing like humans, and is there any merit in living longer but becoming stressed and unhappy?

Severe dieting produces nutrient deficiencies and extreme diets ultimately lead to lowered metabolism, food cravings, over-eating (hyperphagia), depression, poor sleep and many other health problems. Eating, like sleeping, is also part of normal human pleasure.

25... ELECTROMAGNETIC SENSITIVITY

Some people may be sensitive to both natural and man-made electromagnetic fields according to observations and surveys of humans, as well as specific evidence in worms, pigeons and other animals. A US study of electricity workers supported the theory that occupational exposure to electromagnetic fields is associated with an increased risk of suicide.[15] Anything that upsets the nervous system is likely to upset sleep and it is possible that electromagnetic fields from computers and other electronic equipment could be disruptive to the nervous system in various ways.

It has been suggested that powerful magnetic fields are linked to cancer due to a decrease in the body's melatonin levels. (Remember that melatonin is the sleep hormone). However, a study of workers with long-term exposure to 50-Hz magnetic fields indicates no decrease or disruption to melatonin secretion.[16]

My personal and clinical experience is that expensive mattress covers and pillows with small flat magnets in them don't seem to work for insomnia (or anything else?) so buy these as a last resort! There are various magnetic products advertised and they sound great, but the medical sleep centres I contacted, dismissed them and apparently considered they were not worth testing. Nevertheless, there is some research indicating that specific low level emission therapy may improve the sleep of chronic insomniacs.[17]

I have reservations because we are told that fields such as those emitted by mobile phones are potentially harmful while other reports indicate that electromagnetic fields are therapeutic. This implies that the emissions would have to be precisely and individually prescribed. There are reports of people feeling worse from the use of supposed electromagnetic therapy. Until there is more evidence, and equipment proven to work becomes available at a reasonable cost, my suggestions are:

- Try sleeping in a different room or moving the position of the bed. People who are hypersensitive to geomagnetic inlfuences report that they sleep badly if their feet are facing north.

- If you use an electric blanket, heat the bed but turn off the electricity when you turn off the light.

- Don't sleep close to electric appliances such as clock alarms or computers that are still turned on. If you need an alarm to wake you, use a wind up clock.

- Don't sit too close to your TV, and also reduce your watching time.

- Reduce the amount of leisure time spent on the computer.

26... EXERCISE DEFICIENCY

If you don't get adequate daytime physical activity, sleep might not come easily. A trial of people aged 50 to 76 years found that exercise such as low impact aerobics, brisk walking, or stationary cycling, improved sleep quality. [18]

Another study showed that long-term moderate intensity exercise and low intensity stretching improved sleep in women aged between 50 — 75, particularly with those who exercised in the mornings for at least 225 minutes per week.[19] Those who did stretching exercises were less likely to use sleep medication. Those who exercised in the *evenings* for at least 225 minutes per week had *more* trouble falling asleep. Various surveys of people aged over 60 years have confirmed that appropriate exercise therapy is effective. A scientific trial confirms that tai chi enhances sleep in the elderly.[20]

As a yoga teacher I find that the overwhelming majority of evening students are very readily able to physically and mentally relax at the end of 75 minutes exercising although for a few people even yoga exercises are too stimulatory late in the evening.

Generally for insomniacs, exercise needs to be regular, long-term and adequate — and primarily in the early part of the day.

27... EXERCISE EXCESS

At least for poor sleepers, exercising vigorously in the evening is stimulatory and delays sleep. My personal experience is that long hours of physical work at a steady pace is sleep promoting but more than two hours of sustained, vigorous physical exercise daily is over-stimulatory, irrespective of the time of day. While the majority of people say they 'sleep like logs' after a day of skiing or bushwalking, an insomniac may feel physically tired but may sleep poorly.

My suggestion is to have a long 'wind-down' period before

going to bed, particularly if exercising late in the day, and take a magnesium supplement before bed.

28... FEARS

People who have severe, distressing experiences or perceived fears that interfere with their sleep or daytime functioning should seek counselling. There are numerous fears and phobias that can interfere with sleep, including intruders, natural disasters, accidents, insects, diseases, losing your job, terrorists and death. It doesn't help to say that these fears are unfounded because we hear the realities on the news every day, and there's a tiny chance that any one of us could be struck by some calamity. We all have to face the fact that one day we will die and that very few people go through life without injury or a serious illness. I think that having a religious or spiritual belief is the best way of coping with the ups and downs of human life — and the reality that the physical body doesn't last forever.

If you glance through your television guide you will note a plethora of violent shows such as police dramas, war films, medical emergencies, graphic news' photography and animals in distress, so our brains are getting numerous violent imprints without our realizing it. You need to be aware of what's going on around you and in the world, but if you're an insomniac at least be selective in your entertainment.

Fear keeps your brain on the lookout and is linked to light sleep just as in the animal world, the king of the predators (the lion) sleeps about 16 hours a day while fearful prey, such as gazelle, sleep for only a few hours. I'm not saying 'be like a lion' but do all you can to make yourself physically strong, confident and mentally alert, for instance, do a self-defence course, join a church, learn meditation or do a course in self esteem or consult a psychologist.

Bach Flower remedies may help mild cases and the 'anti-fear' remedies include Rock Rose, Mimulus, Aspen and Cherry Plum. Naturopaths and health food stores stock these remedies.

29... FLUID INTAKE, EXCESSIVE OR DEHYDRATION

Excessive fluid intakes will either remain in the body tissues causing pressure and discomfort or will cause excessive urination and mineral loss. Far more people suffer from dehydration or a chronically low fluid intake, and in a hot country such as Australia this problem is very common. Inadequate fluid intake will cause dry mouth, constipation, fatigue, poor mental function, headaches, kidney and metabolic problems.

Appropriate fluid intake depends on your bodyweight, level of activity, temperature, sweating, and your diet and health status. The thirst control centre in our brains may not always work effectively and I see many people who have an inappropriate fluid intake. A 50 kg elderly female with a typical diet and lifestyle and no major medical problems requires around eight glasses of fluid daily — excluding coffee and alcohol. A 90 kg bricklayer working in the heat all day requires many liters of fluid daily. A high protein diet should be accompanied by more fluid than a diet high in fruit and vegetables. If you have disorders of the kidneys or heart, or diabetes your doctor should guide you to drink a specific quantity of fluid daily.

Fluid intake is best spread throughout the day and the recommendation to drink eight glasses of water daily is a general guideline only!

30... GENETIC INFLUENCES

Researchers have found evidence for genetic influences in a number of different sleep disturbances that are distinct from environmental factors, so it's worthwhile checking your family history.

However, we may also inherit bad habits which we can change even though we can't yet change our genes!

31... HEART AND CIRCULATORY DISEASES

Heart problems and/or high blood pressure may cause breathing problems, as well as palpitations, that are more noticeable and stressful when lying flat in bed in a quiet environment. See a cardiologist for all heart problems, lose weight if needed and improve your diet and lifestyle. Even minor degrees of heart failure can interfere with sleep and this problem can be effectively treated by a specialist, so make sure that you get a thorough check up. Some patients find they feel more comfortable if they avoid lying on their left side in bed because this seems to make your heart work harder or at least more noticeably. Magnesium supplementation can help to lower blood pressure and prevent palpitations.

32... HERBAL STIMULANTS AND TONICS

Vitamin B, ginseng and various tonic herbs such as guarana may be very helpful for fatigue, but I always recommend they be taken in the morning. Sensitive insomniacs may find that any type of tonic or nutrient supplement seems to worsen insomnia if taken in the afternoon or evening.

33... HORMONE IMBALANCES

Hormone imbalances play a major role in sleep problems. The hypothalamus is the primary controller or modifier of many hormones, and also modulates body heat, thirst, appetite and other important functions.

Adrenal Stress Hormones

Researchers confirm that people with long-term insomnia have increased blood levels of the adrenal gland stress hormones such as cortisol when measured over a 24-hour period.[21] This means that rather than being anxious about sleep, your hormonal imbalances keep you in a constant state of arousal.

Insomniacs have higher levels of cortisol, particularly in the evening and even during sleep. Typically, a person in this state is an 'owl' (evening type), with bed resistance, generally energetic, competitive, 'nervous' and easily excited but often tired in the mornings. Eventually, most 'owls' become exhausted but still remain somewhat jittery.

To correct this over-arousal, you need a lifestyle that has some routine and calmness and a long, diversionary winding down period before sleep. I recommend a yoga routine every day and also calming herbs (see Chapter 4) and massage or acupuncture. In most cases physical activity early in the day is helpful to settle down the nerves and work off agitation. Before bed you could try taking one level teaspoon of calcium ascorbate powder mixed into a few tablespoons of plain yoghurt and 2 to 4 tablets of magnesium complete to strengthen your adrenal glands.

Where insomniacs are unable to fall asleep before 2 to 3 a.m. it has been demonstrated that 3 to 5 mg of melatonin at 10 p.m. brings forward the sleeping time by about 1½ hours.[22] Melatonin supplementation may have the effect of lowering sleep requirement as a consequence of improved sleep quality. More about melatonin is given in Chapter 5.

Meditation has a calming effect but some aroused people need a system that incorporates mental activity, such as repeating a verse together with visualization, and at the beginning they may be able to concentrate on the meditation technique for a few minutes only.

Growth Hormone

Middle aged adults have less deep slow wave sleep and more light sleep and this is paralleled by a major decline in growth hormone production.[23] Growth hormone regulates body growth, repair and metabolism and has anti-ageing effects. Generally speaking growth hormone therapy is available only for specific medical conditions although it is increasingly used by doctors who specialize in anti-ageing medicine. Growth hormone is expensive and must be given by injection to be really effective. Although it can have miraculous effects it is usually only affordable for the rich and excessive amounts may cause adverse effects, including swelling of arms and legs, joint pain and high blood insulin levels.

The average 60 year old sleeps 30 minutes less every 24 hours compared to a younger person, so as we age we need to work on developing positive thinking and healthy attitudes since we are going to be conscious of our bodies and thoughts for longer periods each day!

Thyroid Hormones

There are many types of thyroid disorders and they all need a medical diagnosis. If thyroid activity is excessive, the main signs are agitation, restlessness, weight loss, fast heartbeat, sweats, tremors and inability to sleep. The symptoms of underactive thyroid include fatigue, weight gain, fluid retention, cold intolerance, mental slowing and excessive or poor sleep. People with low thyroid activity are at risk of snoring and sleep apnoea, which further increases fatigue. A routine medical blood test will accurately detect thyroid abnormalities. I also recommend you take your body temperature in the mornings before you get out of bed; this is called the basal body temperature and measures the temperature in the resting state. If your basal body temperature is consistently less than 36^0 C, this is highly suggestive of an underactive thyroid gland, and this could be responsible for very poor health as well as insomnia. Thankfully, thyroid problems are easily treated with thyroid hormone supplements and the mineral selenium. For more information on thyroid problems, see my book *"Don't Let Your Hormones Ruin Your Life"*

Sex Hormones

Fluctuating or deficient levels of the sex hormones oestrogen and progesterone may cause mood changes in younger females and lead to bouts of poor sleeping. These problems often occur pre-menstrually or after childbirth. I have found that the use of natural progesterone in the form of a cream, capsule or lozenges in a dose of 20 to 75mg daily can greatly reduce these problems. You will need a doctor's prescription for natural progesterone because it is a real hormone and not a herb.

When menopause arrives the body's production of oestrogen and progesterone plummets to very low levels and this can occur gradually or suddenly and is often heralded by inability to sleep.

Although conventional Hormone Replacement Therapy (HRT) is controversial and not without danger, many women report that HRT reduces nocturnal flushing, heat and sweating and settles them down at night. If you are one of those women who cannot sleep without any form of HRT, my personal preference is to prescribe forms of oestrogen and progesterone that are absorbed through the skin and not taken orally. Hormones that are absorbed through the skin are called "transdermal hormones" and pass directly through the skin into the blood circulation, thereby avoiding the liver; thus smaller doses can be used. Suitable forms of transdermal hormones are the creams and patches, both requiring a doctor's prescription. I have found that once the sleep is restored and body temperature settles down, often only very small doses of hormones are required. For more information see my book *"HRT – The Real Truth – Balance your hormones naturally and swing from the chandeliers!"* In a lot of menopausal women, natural menopause formulas such as Femmephase or Promensil which contain phyto-estrogens, along with dietary changes such as increasing legumes, sprouts and ground flaxseeds, will work very well so that HRT is not required.

Low testosterone is linked to sleep disorders in men, notably those who are obese and have obstructive sleep apnea.[24] An exercise program, low carbohydrate eating plan and a liver tonic often work well in such cases. If blood tests show that the abnormally low levels of testosterone persist, a cream containing natural testosterone can be effective, and will usually greatly improve the libido!

Caution: You should take hormones only if they are medically prescribed, and take the lowest therapeutic dose of natural rather than synthetic hormones. Some conditions are treatable only with appropriate hormone replacement therapy but buying hormone remedies via the Internet is neither a sensible or safe option. Using natural means of adjusting hormones, such as herbal medicine, generally takes at least two or three months and these treatments are more successful with practitioner supervision.

34... IMMUNE DYSFUNCTION

Immune compounds (cytokines) in your body alert your brain to inflammation and this in turn alters sleep patterns. Inflammation tends to decrease both slow wave and REM sleep.[25] This reinforces my recommendation to get help for pain and inflammatory disorders, because nothing in your body works in isolation.

Sleep is known to improve the body's reaction to viruses.[26] This explains why you may feel very tired when you have a viral infection, as this is nature's way of telling you to rest. It may also explain why some people feel chronically tired following a bout of the flu or glandular fever — particularly if they didn't rest while they were sick. Perhaps practitioners should prescribe sleep for viral infections rather than giving remedies that allow you to 'soldier on' but jeopardise your wellbeing?

35... ITCHING SKIN

An itchy skin is a common and very distressing cause of poor sleep.

Itching skin may be caused by-

•Immune dysfunction

•Hidden and undiagnosed forms of cancer

•Liver dysfunction such as fatty liver or toxic overload

•Allergies

•Side effects of prescribed medications

•Insects and parasites such as fleas, bites, bed bugs or bird mites

•Excess heat

•Dry skin

•Nervous dermatitis caused by stress and anger

•Skin diseases

See a skin specialist and remove or treat the cause. Although scratching tends to create more inflammation, it's useless to tell people not to scratch because scratching is basically an instinctive reaction. Applying external remedies such as castor oil or a good moisturizer may be soothing or relieving. Successful treatment usually requires lifestyle and dietary changes and improving liver function. I recommend raw juicing, supplements of essential fatty acids (fish oil & flaxseed oil), zinc and selenium and taking a good liver tonic. Check the medications that you are taking as these could be upsetting your liver and/or actually causing the skin condition.

36... JET LAG

Long flights may cause disturbed sleep, fatigue, moodiness, disorientation, and lack of concentration; this is because your biological sleep clock is out of sync with the new time zone you are in. It may take a few days or some weeks for the body to adjust to the new locality. Sometimes you may feel worse during the second or third day after your arrival. Physically fit young people tend to handle changing time zones more effectively.

Suggestions for reducing jet lag:

Before the trip

•Before departure find out the destination arrival times. It is harder for the body to adjust if there is an advance in local time (phase advance), that is, if the new time zone brings forward your bedtime — because you may be able to advance your circadian clock two to three hours only.[27] In other words, it's easier for your body if the new time zone delays your bedtime, which means that travelling westward on a flight from Australia is less confusing for your body clock than an eastward trip.

- Can you plan a more suitable departure and arrival time or perhaps a stopover in a quiet, comfortable place? Your travel agent should be able to help you.

- Cut back on your caffeine and alcohol and anything that might cause withdrawal effects.

- Buy an eye mask and earplugs as you might be sitting close to 'owls', 'readers' and 'snorers' and these inexpensive items may be useful also at your destination. I take a small, battery-operated radio cassette player with some of my own cassettes for the trip — together with earphones — so that I can blot out other noises if necessary.

- Wear loose, comfortable clothing for the trip. Your comfort and circulation will be impeded if you wear tight clothes.

- To keep the blood thin, I usually take one aspirin the day before the flight, one before boarding and one during the flight (all with food) but you should check with your practitioner if you are taking medication or have a health problem.

- Get medical advice if you are on any prescription pharmaceutical. If you get a different prescription or a natural remedy, test it for at least a few days before the flight — in case you have an adverse or unwanted reaction. Generally, sedatives are not recommended because you may not wake adequately if there is an emergency.

During the flight

- Change your watch to coincide with the destination. If possible, plan your sleep to coincide with the normal sleeping time at your destination.

- Avoid alcohol, coffee and carbonated or cola drinks. If you're a heavy user you might have a small quantity to avoid headaches and withdrawal effects but avoid this 3 — 4 hours before your planned sleeping time. Alcohol worsens jet lag and excess can spoil the journey for other passengers.

•Drink plenty of water and some fruit juice because the air inside the plane is dry. Eat lightly. Use a pillow or an inflatable neck collar to get as comfortable as possible.

•Do not eat or drink anything 'new' on the flight to avoid adverse reactions.

•Get up and walk regularly and do some feet and leg exercises whilst sitting.

• Travel first class if you can afford it!

On arrival

•At the destination have some gentle exercise such as walking or yoga to get your muscles stretched and the circulation moving freely, and to help adjust to the tempo of the new location. Have a shower and a nonalcoholic drink.

•If you need to sleep during the day, limit this to a maximum of two hours and set the alarm clock to awaken you.

•Get outdoors in the daylight to help reset your biological sleep clock.

•Have some exercise for the first few days, preferably outdoors and in the morning, to help speed up the adaptation to the new time zone.[28]

•Melatonin may help if taken one hour before bed at a dose of about 3 mg on the first night at the new destination and it may help to continue the melatonin for a week after arrival. A study of professional soccer players indicated that 3 mg melatonin (along with an appropriate light exercise schedule) helped overcome the consequences of jet lag.[29] Do *not* take melatonin *before* the trip because this may worsen jet lag. More details about melatonin are given in Chapter 5.

Future travel may be even harder on our biological rhythm and I see many people in my clinic who are ill following trips to exotic places. One study suggests that space missions lasting more than three months might result in decreased circadian influence and consequent sleep problems.[30] NASA scientists involved with the Mars rover mission had to adjust their schedules to Mars' time, because the rotation of that planet is 39 minutes 35 seconds longer than earth's rotation. Sleep experts gave the scientists advice about light exposure to help them adjust.

37... LIGHT AND DARK EXCESSES
OR INSUFFICIENCIES

Appropriate levels of light and darkness are required for healthful sleep, at least for poor sleepers.

If you have trouble getting to sleep, avoid bright evening lighting and take steps to make your bedroom as dark as possible by using blinds, heavy curtains that are longer and wider than the windows, and perhaps have shutters installed. However, the natural waking process is triggered by the dawn light so if you wake 'groggy' or irritable it may help to have some gentle, early morning light filtering into the bedroom. As soon as you are out of bed open all the blinds and curtains in the house. In Australia, outdoor light is very bright even in winter and the best light therapy is obtained outdoors. The morning light is a strong signal activating your biological clock, and the evening darkness is a signal activating the sleep hormone, melatonin. This is why during winter where the onset of darkness is much earlier it is far better to get to bed earlier than during summer. Many people feel better in the winter because they sleep longer.

Exercise promotes healthful sleep so why not combine physical activity and nature's light therapy? The physical, mental and spiritual benefits of outdoor early morning activity have been promoted for thousands of years and modern surveys have confirmed these benefits. Perhaps the oldest therapeutic exercise is the 12-step yoga sequence 'salute to the sun' (surya namaskar) that was practised by ancient Indian sages at sunrise — and is still part of the early morning routine of many people throughout the world. In the ancient Sanskrit language the sun is expressed by twelve different words and these were chanted in conjunction with the exercise. The sun has been linked to health in many cultures; for example, Hippocrates, the father of modern European medicine, prescribed sunlight and fresh air for a number of illnesses.

The current message in Australia is cover up and avoid the sun — although I recommend early morning outdoor light for my patients. Some researchers say that morning light therapy depends on the light actually entering the eyes and therefore you need to remove contacts and glasses. However, when you are walking towards the early morning sun this light may be irritating to your eyes, so you may need to use sunglasses for *part* of your early morning light exposure. If you are worried about skin cancer or eyestrain, discuss this with your practitioner.

Lux is a measurement of light:

- Common indoor lights are between 300 — 500 lux.
- Light boxes (used for therapeutic purposes in the USA and in some European countries) are typically between 2,500 — 12,000 lux.
- Outdoors on a sunny summer day is about 100,000 lux.
- Full moonlight is about 5 lux.
- A dull, early morning light may be around 3,000 lux.

Experimentally, it has been shown that 1,250 lux can affect human biological rhythm, which means that in the absence of outdoor light you would need to use very bright indoor lighting to change your circadian clock and melatonin levels.

If you require a night light in a hallway, then it is suggested you use red light because this is less disruptive to your sleeping pattern than white or blue light. Putting on the bedside light during the night might completely block melatonin production, and may even disrupt the biological clock of a sleeping bed partner.

Eye masks are readily available and are helpful for people whose partners read in bed. Some of my patients report that their sleep is markedly improved when they use an eye mask.

Appropriate changes in indoor lighting to mimic a normal day may be helpful for shift workers and when travelling between different time zones. Japanese researchers report that elderly nursing home residents have lower melatonin levels because they are inside in a relatively dark environment, however, when they are exposed to bright indoor light for four hours in the middle of the day they have improved sleep.[31]

My own natural light therapy involves getting outside in the morning for 30 — 45 minutes, preferably before 7 a.m. I suggest that you wear shorts and a sleeveless top because there *may* be light receptors on various parts of the body. Sunscreens prevent most of the skin's production of vitamin D that is essential for functioning of bones, muscles and brain. Unfiltered sunlight is more effective for insomniacs and in addition this will allow the body to produce vitamin D.

For patients who wake very early and can't get back to sleep, exposure to evening light might shift the pattern. Remember that the average adult sleeps about seven hours a night and if you go to bed early you will wake early.

Light boxes

Light boxes (phototherapy) are used in some northern countries to treat seasonal affective disorder (winter depression), to normalize the body's biological clock and to help relieve insomnia. Sessions may last for 10 minutes initially and subsequently up to one hour.

There are various types of light therapy equipment including a visor that is worn around the crown of the head and a dawn simulator that mimics the sunrise.[32] I could not find an Australian supplier of light boxes and the two Australian sleep centres I contacted did not recommend light boxes for insomnia.

Cautions using light boxes - If you buy a light box from overseas it should have a diffusing screen that prevents you seeing the contour of the light bulbs and a filter that blocks ultraviolet rays. The field of light should be white and large enough for you to perform sedentary activities while remaining in the light.

People with mania or mood swings may experience excessive mood elevation, and various other side effects of light boxes, have been reported including sunburn, eye problems and headaches.

A feasible option to light boxes is to buy some full-spectrum fluorescent tubes from your hardware store and use these in the house when you first get out of bed, but don't use these particular lights before bedtime.

38... MODERN LIFE

Although modern civilization is much more pleasurable than prehistoric times, our genes have presumably remained more or less unchanged for thousands of years. Our prehistoric ancestors presumably rose when the sun came up and once the sunset, they probably sat around a fire for a while, talked and then went to sleep. About 2700 years ago, the sage in the *Brihadaranyaka Upanishad* described the natural progression from sunlight, to moonlight, to firelight and then to voice. This seems to be a sensible way to settle yourself down for the night and perhaps explains the traditional use of lullabies and story telling — and why I find that audio disks are often effective as a treatment for insomnia.

Now we live in cities that never sleep and at night we are bombarded with lights, electromagnetic fields, news from all over the world and all sorts of stimulating entertainment.

Do you drive to work, habitually skip breakfast, sit at a desk all day, have a sandwich and coffee while working, and return home after sunset?

Do you look at stimulating or disturbing programs on TV or sit at your computer, eat a large meal and have some alcohol?

Why are you surprised that your brain is still 'racing' late into the night when you are trying to sleep?

Working at a frenetic pace from dawn to late evening results in your body producing a high level of stress hormones and these could build up to such a level that restorative sleep is jeopardized. You are probably tired and irritable simply because you don't get adequate sleep!

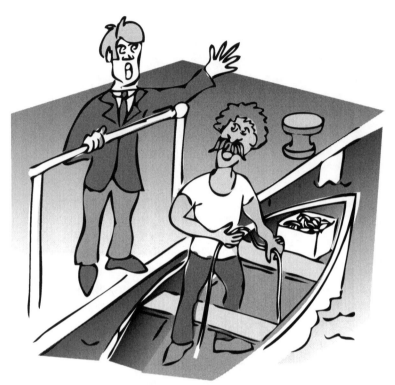

The Good Life - An American businessman was at the pier of a remote coastal village in Mexico when a small boat with just one fisherman docked. In the boat were several kilograms of wonderful shrimp. The American complimented the Mexican on the quality of his shrimp and asked how long it took to catch them. The Mexican replied, 'Only a couple of hours.' The American then asked why he didn't stay out longer and catch more? The Mexican said he had enough to support his family's immediate needs.

The American enquired, 'But what do you do with the rest of your time?' The Mexican replied, 'I sleep late, fish a little, play with my children, take siesta with my wife, Maria, stroll into the village each evening where I have a few drinks and play guitar with my amigos. I have a full and busy life, senor.' The American scoffed, 'I have a business degree from Harvard University and can advise you. You should spend more time shrimping and with the money buy a bigger boat. With the proceeds from the bigger boat you could buy several boats; eventually you would have a fleet of fishing boats. Instead of selling your catch to a middleman you would sell directly to the processor, eventually opening your own cannery. You would need to leave this small coastal village and move to Mexico City. Then you would move to Los Angeles and eventually to New York — where you will run your expanding enterprise.'

The Mexican fisherman asked, 'But senor, how long with this take?' To which the American replied, 'Fifteen to twenty years.' 'But what then, senor?' The American laughed and said, 'That's the best part. When the time is right you would set up a company and sell shares to the public. You would become very rich; you would make millions.' 'Millions, senor. Then what?' The American said, 'Then you could retire; move to a small coastal fishing village, where you could sleep late, fish a little, play with your grandchildren, take siesta with your wife, stroll to the village in the evenings where you would have a few drinks and play guitar with your amigos.'   *Anonymous*

39... MOUTH BREATHING
(NASAL, SINUS OR RESPIRATORY CONGESTION)

The most common cause of mouth breathing is congestion or obstruction in the nasal passages, adenoids or the sinuses. This is most commonly due to deviation of the nasal septum, inhalant allergies and/or infections. Consult a specialist ear nose and throat doctor to check this out. In severe cases treatments may demand surgery, antihistamines and even a short course of antibiotics and nasal steroids. However in the long term you will need to turn to natural therapies to achieve success. Some basic suggestions for natural remedies are given in Chapter 5.

40... NEUROLOGICAL DISEASES

Many parts of the brain are involved in the sleep process so various degenerative diseases of the brain are likely to interfere with sleep. For instance poor sleep and daytime fatigue, as well as parasomnias (such as vigorous movements during REM sleep), may precede Parkinson's disease by some years.[33]

People with Alzheimer's disease and related dementias frequently have sleep problems including nighttime agitation, decreased REM sleep, and excessive daytime napping.[34] If these diseases are suspected please see a neurologist who will perform a CAT scan or an MRI scan.

41... NIGHTMARES AND DISTURBING DREAMS

When you dream your brain sees, hears, and participates in activities that are not there. The dreams may be so lifelike that they awaken you, sometimes with a startle. Dreaming sleep (REM) takes up about 20 per cent of total sleeping time and humans start dreaming as a foetus in the uterus.

A traumatic event may cause recurring nightmares and the event may be re-experienced many times during sleep as part of post traumatic stress syndrome. Frequent nightmares may also occur in the absence of any trauma. Adults who are lifelong nightmare sufferers may have features of schizophrenia but are generally sensitive, artistic and creative.[35]

All our experiences are woven into the brain and the way our brain sorts out the events may manifest as a 'scrambled' dream, and therefore we should not be concerned unless dreams frequently prevent sleep and cause daytime fatigue.

Anxious dreams may be caused by stressful intellectual activity, such as being told you have to complete an exam within a certain time and achieve a specific, high mark. When dreams are perturbing this may be a reflection of a current worry or caused by drugs and diseases — such as Parkinson's. However, vivid dreamers do not appear to have a different psychological profile from dreamers.

An ancient Indian sage considered that the dreaming state was when man's ordinary self becomes his spiritual self. In other words, dreaming allows your soul to experience events just as you might enjoy a dramatic film.

> *After enjoying himself and roaming in the dream state*
> *And merely seeing the effects of merits and demerits*
> *He comes back to his former condition, the waking state*
> *Brihadaranyaka Upanishad, IV.iii.35*

Nightmares and dreams may be "neurological junk", unconscious desires, expressions of anxiety, responses to magnetic fields, symbolic messages, manifestations of guilt, or even spiritual experiences. Various scientific experts and psychologists have attempted to interpret dreams but dreams are probably beyond the realm of science. When four psychoanalysts were given details about a particular dream, they all had different ideas about the meaning of that dream.[36]

Since we can't control dreams, my advice is not to worry unduly about them. Although we are fascinated by our own dreams, if you observe your 'listeners' carefully you will see that most people are not at all interested in hearing a detailed account of *your* dreams. If nightmares or upsetting dreams frequently disturb your sleep, consult a qualified psychologist.

42... NIGHT SWEATS

Night sweats may be linked to fevers caused by infections or inflammation. The infection may be hidden or not clinically apparent to you or your doctor; for example it may be hidden in the sinuses, teeth, gums, intestines or lungs. This is why it is important to see a diagnostic physician if you have persistent night sweats and over heating associated with poor health for no apparent reason. Get a deep and thorough check up before it's too late!

Aim to find the cause and this may require blood and urine tests and CAT scans to check for infections, the status of your immune system and your liver.

Overheating and sweating may be caused by liver disorders, such as fatty liver or chronic hepatitis, and improving liver function is often very effective in removing overheating and night sweats. I recommend a good liver tonic and raw juicing using purple cabbage, ginger root, carrot, beetroot, orange and green leafy vegetables. It is easy to check the health of your liver with a simple ultrasound scan of the abdomen and a blood test to check liver enzymes.

Night sweats and/or overheating in mature aged women who are otherwise well and fit are usually caused by the oestrogen deficiency of the menopause. For information on menopause see page 67.

One memorable patient of mine was a middle-aged woman who complained that sweating at night kept her awake. When I questioned her about blankets she told me that she didn't use blankets and as an afterthought added that she used a lightweight doona. I saw her in Sydney in January! My advice was to put the doona in a cupboard until May but she insisted it was lightweight and not the cause of the problem. I pointed out that in cold countries in winter, a lightweight doona is often the only bedcover because it generates and retains heat. For some children, and adults, excess bed covers apparently provide them with a feeling of security and they are reluctant to give them up.

43... NOCTURNAL MYOCLONUS (MUSCLE CONTRACTIONS)

These are not the 'normal' jerking movements that sometimes occur as we are falling to sleep but are more prolonged and severe jerking movements that prevent sleep throughout the night. Regular exercise and supplementation with the mineral magnesium and the amino acid taurine may help a lot. Work with your practitioner to find the right dose, as often high doses are needed. If symptoms persist see a neurologist to exclude neurological disorders like Multiple Sclerosis or Parkinson's disease.

44... NOISE

Some people are very sensitive to noise in general or to particular noises. For instance, a dripping tap or a ticking clock is torture, but the sound of rain on a tin roof is often soothing. Your own dog's bark may be cute or reassuring but a neighbor's barking dog is irritating noise pollution.

If your neighbors are entertainers, chefs or shift workers, you have to understand that they are entitled to live a normal life in their free time. And, others may not want to coordinate their lives to your bedtime. Although we should be neighborly, there are laws about excessive noise levels and if there is an unreasonable noise that repeatedly disrupts your sleep there are various steps you can take:

1. Change your perception of the noise. Do you go to bed and wait anxiously for the irritating sound? It is not possible for poor sleepers to block out irritating sounds; instead think that the noise is washing over you, or imagine that the sound is from a different source. For instance, a barking dog is a cute little puppy. Imagine the puppy, what type is it, what color, and so on — try to picture every detail.

2. Use earplugs that you can buy over-the-counter at most pharmacies. You may have to try a few different types, and generally these deaden

the noise rather than obliterate it completely but still they can be extremely effective. Some people find earplugs adequately reduce the sound of snoring.

3. If it's an outside noise, perhaps have double windows or shutters for your bedroom. If you are desperate you can even have the bedroom sound-proofed. I've been told that corkboard about 2.5 cm thick is effective!

4. Use some pleasant music, relaxation or meditation tapes or audio books to mask unwanted sounds. 'White noise' such as the hum of an air conditioner can block out other noises. If you are noise sensitive you may find that even neutral sounds, such as air conditioners, are disturbing, in which case you may be able to imagine that you are resting comfortably in a soft green rain forest listening to the sounds of the breeze in the canopy as you visualize the details of the forest. I 'think' that my cooling fan sounds like rain. Sometimes absence of noise keeps people awake! City dwellers, for instance, may experience that they can't sleep without the familiar sound of traffic.

5. *Wait* until you're feeling calm and speak to the offender. Simply explain that the problem noise disturbs your sleep. *This is a last resort* as most 'noisy' people are inconsiderate and will get angry, irrespective of how you approach them and they may deliberately increase the noise or become more of a nuisance in other ways — or tell you about some of your irritating habits. If the noise is unreasonable, and your friendly request is ignored, contact your local council to find out the regulations. You'll be surprised to learn, for instance, how high the fines can be for barking dogs and there are limits to *all* noise, based on the decibel level above normal background noise, at your property boundary.

45... OBESITY

As you will see in this chapter under 'apnoea' and 'snoring', excess body weight may be a big impediment to sleeping. Excess weight may cause nighttime urination, reflux of stomach acid, shallow breathing, overheating and sweating. Obesity may cause changes in total slow wave sleep, as well as changes in switching to and from the different categories of sleep[37] and daytime fatigue is the likely outcome.

For a powerful and delicious low carbohydrate eating plan to lose weight safely see chapter 23 in my book titled *"Can't Lose Weight? You could have Syndrome X – the chemical imbalance that makes your body store fat"*

Syndrome X is the most common cause of being overweight and it is associated with high levels of the hormone insulin, which is a fat-storing hormone and also causes fatty liver. Syndrome X sufferers often have sleep problems such as overheating and sleep apnoea. My program effectively reduces insulin levels and changes your metabolism from fat storing into fat burning. Syndrome X often leads to diabetes type 2 so the earlier you reverse it the better.

46...OVERWORK

If your job demands that you get up early, then you simply have to go to bed relatively early. No one should be so indispensable that they do not have time to get a reasonable night's sleep. There's a Zen story about a man on horseback. The horse is galloping and someone yells to the rider, 'Where are you going?' The rider shouts back 'I don't know, but the horse does.' Some of us are going flat out for no sound reason and in some situations it's like a stampede and the whole office or the whole family is pushed into excess activity and insufficient sleep.

A few people are indispensable, such as mothers with young children and carers — and if you're in this category try to nap during the day and do all you can to get others to take some of the workload and responsibility. My sister Madeleine had this problem in the 1980s and her huge workload as a mother of 3 young children and a carer of her elderly father almost caused her to have a stress breakdown. Madeleine narrowly averted this "nervous breakdown" or stress breakdown by a combination of her own mental therapy and using a very small dose of a sleeping tablet. After six nights of not sleeping at all and not having enough relatives nearby to help her, she felt she was about to have a nervous collapse and thus would be unable to care for anyone including herself.

Madeleine decided upon two things –

1. She would stop listening to her mind that was telling her by 4 p.m. each day that she was not going to be able to sleep that night

2. Although she was committed to a healthy lifestyle and took heaps of vitamins, she would take a sleeping tablet to help her get through the crisis, which was going to last another 6 months.

Madeleine visited her local doctor and asked for a sleeping tablet. She took half a tablet and it worked like a charm and she narrowly averted a stress breakdown. After one week she found that all she needed to take was one quarter of a sleeping tablet. This worked for Madeleine because she had trouble falling off to sleep because of her huge work load and stress level, and once asleep she had no trouble staying asleep. This strategy will not work for everyone who is overloaded to the point of a stress breakdown, but I thought it was an interesting case history for those who have got to the point where "the last straw breaks the camel's back." Don't wait until it's too late and you have a stress breakdown – make your self heard and get help!

47... PAIN AND STIFFNESS

You've probably heard people say that arthritis and other painful joint problems are worse at night. I always thought that this was because the mind was not distracted by other things. However, inflammatory cytokine compounds are produced by the body in higher quantities during the night and early morning while the body's adrenal cortisol and ACTH levels are typically relatively low.[38] These findings may partly explain the morning stiffness experienced by most arthritis sufferers.

Headaches, sore neck, tight shoulders, aching feet, intestinal colic and anything that causes pain or prevents relaxation of the body is likely to be linked to poor sleeping. Try yoga or tai chi, join the local gym, start swimming and have a regular massage (for more information on natural remedies see page 42).

It is known, for example, that fibromyalgia sufferers have somewhat different brain wave patterns during sleep and this may explain why the condition is linked to non-restorative sleep and consequent fatigue.

Get professional help and do all you can to reduce pain because pain can cause more inflammation and, unless you're super-human, pain can also lead to fatigue and depression. Don't listen to those who tell you that pharmaceuticals are the only treatment but don't be a pain martyr either! Some pain definitely needs pharmaceuticals.

48... PETS

The Mayo Clinic Sleep Disorders Center, USA, assessed the frequency and severity of sleep disruption caused by family pets. Out of 300 insomnia patients, 52 per cent had one or more pets, mostly cats and dogs. More than half of those pet owners had disrupted sleep every night although only one per cent thought their sleep was disrupted for more than 20 minutes each night on average. Snoring occurred in 21 per cent of dogs and seven per cent of cats. Cats were more likely to be allowed in the bedroom and on the bed.[39] This American report does not mention animals actually in bed but this is even more disruptive.

Pets have an important benefit for those who feel insecure because dogs, cats and other animals often have better sight and smell than humans and they give various warning signals when strangers approach the house or when something unusual happens.

I have a number of patients who habitually lose a lot of sleep because their animals are ill, have lost bladder or bowel control, demand to be fed or patted, or the pets want company while they go outside to look at the stars. Although you may be very attached to animals I don't recommend you have them in the bedroom and this has to start from day one. After all, we don't have our human children sleeping with us all their lives. Animal lovers will generally ignore this advice because they have an emotional need to be close to their pets.

49... PHARMACEUTICALS

A number of pharmaceuticals interfere with normal sleep patterns. A significant REM sleep reduction was shown for 16 of 21 antidepressant pharmaceuticals.[40] Phenelzine, an antidepressant (monoamine oxidase inhibitor) may completely suppress REM sleep.[41] Each of the various stages of sleep is important for physical, mental and emotional wellbeing, and REM sleep specifically helps learning and brain function.

Other pharmaceuticals that may disrupt normal sleep include Catapres, Xanax, theophyline, decongestants, stimulants, diuretics, slimming pills and some hormones such as cortisone. Benzodiazepines, commonly prescribed for insomnia and anxiety, reduce the pineal gland's production of melatonin.[42]

Beta-blockers (prescribed mainly for hypertension) inhibit melatonin production. Ventolin may cause agitation in sensitive adults and children.

Many pharmaceuticals including over-the-counter antihistamines, have the potential to upset your nervous system. Some pharmaceuticals can cause rebound effects or withdrawal symptoms, including insomnia. If you suspect a problem with any medication or natural remedy contact the practitioner who prescribed the medication, or the person who sold the product to you, and let your doctor know.

50... PHYSICAL DISCOMFORT

Hot feet, abdominal bloating, cramps and blocked nose are examples of factors that are likely to impede sleep. If you have a problem that is not corrected or alleviated by your own efforts, get practitioner help because not everything corrects itself with time and one problem can lead to another.

Your environment, sleeping position and mattress are also important for restorative sleep and these topics are covered in this chapter. It's surprising that insomniacs often pay little practical attention to their nighttime comfort but they worry about everything.

51... PSYCHIATRIC DISORDERS

Mental illnesses are a common cause of insomnia and are accompanied by deficits in brain wave patterns during sleep. Depression is commonly associated with waking during the night or very early in the morning and not being able to get back to sleep. These are generalizations because, for example, some depressed patients may sleep excessively.

Schizophrenia and the manic phases of manic-depressive illness are associated with inability to get off to sleep.

Psychiatric disorders require the care of a psychiatrist so that the patients and their families can function in reasonable harmony. Some advice in this book would *not* be appropriate for self-treatment of psychiatric disorders, such as relying on natural remedies or light-box therapy, but getting some early morning outdoor activity and avoiding excess coffee and junk food is beneficial for everyone.

52... PSYCHOLOGICAL STRESS

If you lie in bed vainly trying to sleep or focusing on your problems, this causes increased anxiety and frustration that will ultimately lead to signs of physical stress.

•Adrenalin and glucose are released into your blood, your heartbeat quickens, blood pressure rises and your body is geared for 'fight or flight'.

•Your hearing and other senses become more sensitive.

•Teeth grinding occurs quite commonly in stressed teenagers and adults, and a mouth guard or dental work may be required to prevent damage to teeth and jaws.

I sometimes see elderly people who are badgered by their children for not grieving 'appropriately' over someone who died decades ago. The grown-up children have read somewhere that you need 'closure' or some specific grieving process to recover, but this is not necessarily so. Reactivating memories may reactivate the problem because the parent is constantly being reminded of the past sad event and may even feel guilty about not responding or behaving in a particular way. Other patients I see are still clearly angry over a perceived insult that occurred decades ago.

You can change the way you handle stress and pressure and this involves awareness of your thinking and behavior:

• Are your demands on yourself (and others) excessive and do you take the time to get a balance of sleep, fun, work, learning, eating properly — and doing nothing in particular. Some patients tell me that they don't have time to eat properly and others are working such long hours they don't have time to get adequate sleep. If you have an ongoing problem there are only three courses open to you: get help, change the situation, or accept it and find compensations.

• Learn to say 'no' in a tactful way when asked to do more. You can't help everyone and everything. Perhaps do a course in assertiveness or self esteem.

• Learn to say 'yes' when people tell you to take a break. Plan mini-breaks to prevent a build up of chain reactions in your body and mind. Go outside and play with the kids; take a walk in the park in your lunch break, schedule regular physical activity and go outside at night to look at the stars! When did you last have a long, leisurely meal, enjoying the food and the company, and chatting about nothing in particular?

• Spend five minutes every day focusing on your breathing. As you breathe out, imagine you are breathing out grey smoke and that smoke represents your worries and negative thoughts. Feel that you are getting rid of anything that you don't want or don't need. You can do this visualization exercise while travelling or walking. When your workload seems excessive, remind yourself that you can do only one thing at a time. Make a mental or written list of smaller tasks aiming to focus on your first task rather than the whole list.

•Insomnia is more common in people who live alone, the unemployed, the elderly, and homemakers. Perhaps this indicates that they have less chance to 'talk out' their worries and more time to dwell on them. Laughter, a known antistress therapy, occurs more frequently when you are with others. Getting out of the house, socializing, doing volunteer work, joining a church group, learning new things and joining a walking club may be part of solving insomnia

•Read the Psalms and Proverbs, and you are bound to find some appropriate words that you can silently repeat to help you focus on the present rather than worrying about the past or the uncertain future. Buddhist texts are excellent for teaching mindfulness so you can enjoy the present. Remember, the two main aims of human existence: Firstly, to enjoy it and secondly to find inner peace.

53... RESPIRATORY INFECTIONS AND DISEASES

A number of body functions are reduced during sleep but if anything impedes your breathing your brain will wake you.

Treating the respiratory system with appropriate natural therapies can correct sleeping problems in some adults and children.

Infections such as the common cold make you so uncomfortable that you can't get to sleep, although rest is one of the best antiviral treatments. Coughing is a reflex and part of the body's system to keep your airways clear and that's why practitioners are careful not to overly suppress this action.

Respiratory problems such as asthma, nasal obstructions, bronchitis and bronchiectasis, which are associated with excessive mucous production and nocturnal cough can be improved by the following –

Vitamin C

Fish oil and flaxseed oil

A raw juice containing ginger root, orange, carrot, radish and fenugreek

A dairy free diet

Selenium and zinc which also reduce viral infections

Regular physiotherapy and postural drainage

If you have hay fever, as well as the above, you may need to consider non-allergenic pillows.

See a respiratory physician if the nocturnal cough persists and don't forget that a nocturnal cough can be due to sinus infection or gastric reflux.

54... RESTLESS LEG SYNDROME

It is common for people over 65 years of age to experience periodic limb movements or sensations causing an urge to move their legs, while they are resting or during sleep; this is not a problem unless it makes you feel uncomfortable or is linked to insomnia or daytime sleepiness. However, uncontrollable restlessness of the body or jerking movements of the limbs delays or interrupts sleep. The causes may include dopamine (brain chemical) abnormalities, magnesium deficiency, vitamin D deficiency, deficiencies of essential fatty acids, poor circulation or anaemia due to low levels of iron, folate or vitamin B12.

A study of young people with restless leg syndrome found that they had levels of iron slightly below normal, and oral iron supplementation for four to five months markedly diminished the problem. Do not take iron supplementation unless you have had a blood test verifying that your iron levels are low because iron excess causes health problems.

Another possible cause of restless legs is that the sleeping position may irritate the spinal cord at the area of the lower back affecting the nerve fibres that run down the legs. Refer below under the heading 'sleeping position' for my recommendations and the use of an extra pillow for the legs.

Cramps in the legs are a common cause of insomnia and can be due to poor circulation, diabetes or pre-diabetes (Syndrome X), lack of exercise or magnesium deficiency. You can get aching legs as well as cramps, as a consequence of taking diuretic drugs and laxatives, because they cause urinary and faecal mineral loss.

If you have nocturnal cramps in your limbs you will usually find that taking a supplement of magnesium complete in a dose of 4 tablets daily fixes the problem. Magnesium is generally safe and well tolerated, and as well as preventing the cramps and spasms, it helps to totally relax your nervous system in a natural and safe way. High doses of magnesium can have a laxative effect. I also recommend supplements of fish oil and flaxseed oil along with lecithin to improve the health of the nerves to the muscles.

The father of one of my friends could not sleep because of leg cramps although he slept soundly on Friday nights after his daughter took him to dinner at the local Chinese restaurant. When he added a *little* soy sauce (which is salty) to his evening meals he slept much better.

55... SEIZURES AND SERIOUS BRAIN DISORDERS

This is probably the least common cause of sleep disorders and people with these disorders would experience additional symptoms, indicating that there is an underlying serious problem.

These symptoms could include; frequent headaches, visual problems, major changes in personality, dizziness, weakness or numbness of the limbs and nausea or vomiting.

If you have these problems see your doctor as soon as possible, as you probably need to have an MRI or CAT scan of the brain.

56... SEX DEPRIVATION

Satisfying sex is highly recommended for insomnia but it is not always attainable or available. For most people satisfying sex is linked to agreeable relationships. This involves making time for each other, and for personal wellbeing.

57... SHIFT WORK

Researchers consider that shift workers should be encouraged to adopt a consistent sleep schedule to reduce poor sleep, health problems and accidents.[43] Shift workers need to be aware that they have a higher rate of work-related injuries compared to other workers and that the accident rate is even higher if they have to keep pace with machines.

Circadian adaptation may be helped by bright light during working hours and a darkened bedroom, although the degrees of darkness and light required vary with each individual. Normal nighttime sleep is accompanied by changes in the whole body. For instance, the digestive system slows down during sleep and therefore eating meals at an inappropriate circadian phase may contribute to the higher level of gastrointestinal problems that occurs in shift workers.

One study indicates that melatonin does *not* help *rotating* shift workers.[44] However, melatonin may be helpful for those with permanent night shifts, especially if accompanied by appropriate light and dark exposure, and exercise.

58...SLEEPING POSITION

My recommended sleep position for adult insomniacs is:

•Lie on your right side — because you will be less conscious of your heartbeat. (Listening to your heartbeat may cause anxiety.)

•Use a pillow that supports the natural curvature of the neck (see page 45).

•Bend the left knee so that the left thigh is more or less at right angles. Ideally, have another pillow in front of your body and under the left knee because this will keep your spine aligned and prevent stress on your lower back.

•Ideally the right arm is in front of you, more or less at shoulder level. If you have broad shoulders, your left shoulder and upper body may be tilted somewhat backward. The left arm is slightly bent and to your front. This is basically the same as the 'stable side position' in first aid.

Sleeping on your back encourages mouth breathing, leading to dryness of the mouth and throat, and snoring, and it can be stressful on the lower back unless you place a large pillow under the knees. However, back sleeping is said to be linked to confidence.

Sleeping on your front is stressful for your lower back and neck; and the heart and respiratory system have to work harder. I suggest you gradually retrain yourself to sleep on your side.

Sudden infant death syndrome (SIDS) is outside the scope of this book, however, some Australian researchers advise that sleeping on the stomach is a major risk factor because this impairs heart rate control.[45] Infants with lung problems may breathe easier in this position but in a hospital setting they are continuously monitored. Research papers on SIDS are published continually and your baby health centre or practitioner will keep you informed of any major developments.

If you're a good sleeper and do not disturb others don't bother changing your way of sleeping.

59... SLEEP ROUTINE INSUFFICIENCY

Establishing sleep-enhancing habits by retraining the brain is known as 'sleep hygiene'. There is no absolute agreement about the steps to be applied and the extent to which they should be used.[46] It seems obvious, for instance, that you would not use forms of sleep deprivation on children and that some people find it intensely upsetting to change their habits. My general advice is to change your routines *slowly* because even healthy changes are stressful. An *ideal* strategy is as follows:

1. Get up at the same time every morning, irrespective of your bedtime. The *perfect* waking time is sunrise, and then you should open the blinds letting in as much natural light as possible. Have a drink, and get at least 30 minutes of light physical outdoor activity preferably near greenery or water. There is evidence that this early morning light will help maintain your circadian rhythm. If the low early morning sunlight irritates your eyes, wear sunglasses but only when facing the sun. Early morning light is important because this gives your brain and body the message to set your nighttime sleepiness clock. Initially you are not going to bed earlier so you will be somewhat sleep deprived. Depending on your lifestyle it may be easier to begin getting out of bed 15 or 30 minutes earlier and gradually improving, but do not lie in bed awake for more than about ten minutes once it's daylight because that gives your brain the message that bed is for lolling around, or worrying. Depending on lifestyle and long-term habits I usually recommend getting up before 7 a.m. but it doesn't matter if your retraining takes months or years.

Caution: Elderly people usually need a different protocol because they tend to go to bed earlier and sleep somewhat fewer hours — as discussed in Chapter 1 under the heading 'sleep in the elderly'.

2. Do not nap during the day if you're a poor sleeper unless you are a pilot, shift worker, carer or mother, and are necessarily woken during the night.

3. Keep to the program seven days a week. It may take up to two months for your biological sleep clock to actually change but after a few weeks you may find that you are feeling tired somewhat earlier in the evening.

4. Do not have coffee and other stimulants after lunch.

5. Do not exercise vigorously after dinner.

6. After dinner, do the dishes, clean your teeth, change your clothes, and get the bed prepared. Some sleep experts consider that the 'sleepiness message' comes in cycles every 60 to 90 minutes; therefore, if you begin activities such as washing the dishes when you *start* feeling tired you'll over-ride that message and have to wait another hour or so. (I think my own sleepiness messages come in two-hour cycles and this personal experience reminds me that much information about sleep is averaged, so don't be concerned if you don't match the statistics). In addition, tidy up, get organized for the next day so you don't have to worry about getting out of the house on time the next morning. Some people are punctuality zealots and worry about being late. If you get your clothes out, for example, this will also save time, decision-making and stress in the mornings. In summary, get everything organized early in the evening so you simply have to fall into bed!

7. Do not go to bed until you feel sleepy otherwise you will lie in bed agitating yourself.

8. Rather than worrying about being late the next day, set an alarm clock or organise a phone 'wake-up' call.

9. Don't work too late at night but do something 'distracting' but not too stimulating. Remember that cemeteries are full of indispensable people!

> Consider how falling drops of water fill a jar,
> Just as the wise accomplish merit little by little.'
> Buddha

10. Perhaps have a warm relaxing bath with a few drops of lavender oil in it. More details are given about baths in Chapter 5.

11. If you're in an excited or agitated state, you may need a long winding down or diverting activity before you can relax. Reading and or TV is good for winding down; choose a program that is not upsetting or over stimulating.

12. As a general rule, don't lie in bed 'trying to sleep' for more than 45 minutes. The usual recommendation is to get up and do something. However, I think this recommendation must be made by good sleepers because if you can't sleep you generally feel terrible and you simply don't want to get up. You want to sleep! Furthermore, if you put on a light and start *doing* things, this will give your body and brain the message that the night is for activities. My suggestion is to have a portable audio system next to your bed so that if you wake and can't get back to sleep, you can listen to nice music, interesting radio shows or relaxing audio disks. My recommendations about audio books are given below but you may have to experiment to find out what suits you. Personally I find that music, breathing or relaxation techniques do not sufficiently occupy the brain to divert thoughts. If you wake very early in the morning, then I think it is preferable to get up and begin your day's activity — but it requires great willpower to get out of bed if you're tired! Poor sleepers should not spend more than eight hours in bed because lying in bed in the vain hope of sleeping will aggravate insomnia.

13. Don't have a clock within view because this will upset you if you're having a bad night and if you keep looking at the time. I do not recommend that you keep a sleep diary unless your practitioner suggests this in conjunction with a specific sleep treatment. Writing notes about your sleep — or lack of it — is likely to increase anxiety.

14. During your sleep retraining period, the time in bed may be between five to eight hours, depending on your level of insomnia.

15. The ultimate aim is to get to bed by 10 p.m. and to get up at 6 a.m. but if you work late, a schedule of 11 p.m. to 6.30 — 7 a.m. may be more appropriate.

•If you are continuously going to bed extremely late, a more heroic treatment is to go to bed even later but get up early. Then you will be exhausted and *want* to get to bed early the following night. This works for some people, but be aware that your physical and mental function will be compromised due to sleep deprivation while you are trying to re-set your biological sleep clock.

•Some sleep experts say that you should *not* read in bed, however, I find that reading is an effective sleep inducer. If the reading light upsets your partner, perhaps your partner could use an eye mask. I think that spiritual or travel books are good because they are neither boring nor stimulating and you are not tempted to speed read to find out what happens at the end. My preferences are texts with commentaries of the *Bhagavad Gita* and the *Upanishads*, and any book by the Dalai Lama and Thich Nhat Hanh. Buddhist books usually contain much common sense advice about daily life that is not contrary to any particular religion. You may prefer the Bible or texts related to your own beliefs. There are specialist religious and alternative bookshops in large cities, and most libraries have a reasonable selection (see Appendix I).

•Another option is to read the classics or philosophical books and then at least you can boast that you have actually read them. The trick is to train yourself to read slowly, savoring each word or thought, appreciating the language, rather than speed reading to see if anything exciting pops up. The following is *my* short list:

Don Quixote, by Miguel de Cervantes

Life of Samuel Johnson, by James Boswell

The Magic Mountain, by Thomas Mann

Moby Dick, by Herman Melville

Pilgrim's Progress, by John Bunyan

Remembrance of Things Past, by Marcel Proust

Vanity Fair, by William Makepeace-Thackeray

Free Thinking, by Stephanie Dowrick

Where There's a Will, by John Mortimer

The Road Less Travelled, by Scott Peck

You Can Heal Your Life, by Louise Hayes

These books are readily available in libraries and most book stores.

If you use your eyes all day, you may prefer audio books. Unfortunately, the list of suitable 'nighttime' talking books is relatively limited but some that I have found useful include:

A Year in Provence, by Peter Mayle

The Old Patagonian Express, by Paul Theroux

I make my own cassettes and have recorded for my personal use Eastern philosophical texts such as *The Bhagavad Gita* and *The Dharmapada*. Once you get used to listening to yourself, your own voice becomes familiar and soothing, but you need to do the recording when you're having a 'good day'. Don't attempt to make your reading theatrical but read calmly and slowly in your everyday voice.

Audio books are ideal for people who wake during the night and can't get back to sleep, because all you have to do is press the 'play' switch and say to yourself 'I'm going to listen to each word'. The more I tell myself to listen to the words, the quicker I get back to sleep and now I rarely hear the latter part of the cassettes.

Some relaxation CDs *don't* work for me because they are 'syrupy' and seem to reinforce the notion that I am not feeling relaxed or peaceful. Always listen to at least part of a disk before purchasing because the voice or sounds may not suit you. The actual sound of the voice and a regular pace seems to relax me more than the story, although it is *probably* helpful to have something uplifting for our minds as we drift into sleep. My belief is that appropriate sounds are the best sleep inducers. Your local bookstore and library may be able to help you find CDs and cassettes that appeal to you and I have given a few sources in Appendix I.

Your sleep will be more restorative if your life is reasonably in sync with natural light. Establishing a sleep routine is troublesome but it is worthwhile in the long run and once sleep has improved you will find that you can be somewhat flexible.

60... SNORING

Snoring may or may not be linked to sleep apnoea. Simple (primary) snoring is the noise made by the vibrations of the soft tissues in the throat while breathing in. It may cause others to lose sleep and to lose their tempers, and can lead to loss of friendships and partners. Few people choose to share a bedroom with a snorer.

Snoring may be caused by obesity, excess alcohol, sleeping on the back, exhaustion, how the throat is structured, or respiratory system disorders. Habitual mouth breathing may lead to snoring, and the health advantages of breathing through the nose are covered under 'apnoea' in this chapter. Apart from the fact that snoring may dry the mouth and throat tissues of snorers, it is estimated that the bed partners of snorers lose one hour's sleep a night and this is likely to cause sleep-deprived stress and a higher disease risk for the bed partner.

As far as possible remove the causes of snoring, and refer to Chapter 5 for a basic breathing technique and ways of clearing nasal passages. The snorer's partner could use special earplugs and information about these is given on page 146.

For the snorer, you can buy over-the-counter products from pharmacies and these sometimes reduce the problem. Sewing a tennis ball onto the back of the pyjama top may help because it prevents lying on the back. Other options include dental mouth guards and a strap-like support for the jaw that fits over the top and back of the head and under the chin. You can view this on http://www.quietnitecap.com/nav.html. Sleep apnoea centres supply more complex equipment but before buying equipment discuss this with your practitioner. If you're desperate, surgery and laser treatments are extreme options but they may not be a permanent solution.

> Caution: Snorers generally have 'relaxed' throat tissues and sleeping tablets may make the throat even more relaxed.

61... SPIRITUAL POVERTY

I presume that people who have genuine inner peace are more likely to be relatively good sleepers. An explanation for the common saying 'I had a good sleep' is that when you are in deep sleep you are in God's hands.

Do you ever lie in bed and become aware of an 'uneasy' feeling? Often, if you think through the day's events, that feeling is your conscience letting you know you have done something wrong. One suggestion is that before you go to bed, you sit quietly and mentally observe your actions for that day. Were *your* motives and actions worthy? Be honest, don't blame others and know that the way to improve the world is to improve yourself. Forgive yourself and resolve to do better next day. Silently repeat a few times, 'I forgive myself for any mistakes I have made and I forgive everyone'.

Poor sleepers can lie awake for hours going over some real or unintentional hurt imposed on them and going over how they should have responded — while the person who committed the misdeed is probably sleeping peacefully without a care in the world!

Humans are imperfect. In the same way, your own faith may not be practised perfectly by all followers and leaders, so don't abandon it because of the actions of a few. Changing or losing your 'faith' can be stressful in subtle ways and may result in health problems, including insomnia.

Having a religious belief or developing a spiritual philosophy may be a solution for some insomniacs. If you practice your faith and go to meetings or services with like-minded people, research shows that this type of involvement also improves your physical and mental wellbeing.

Ministers, priests, swamis, monks and other religious teachers undertake spirituality as their full-time job so you should be able to find someone to help answer your questions. There are many wise and noble teachers and if you want to explore your own or other traditions always take your 'sensible self' with you. Spiritual teachers are there to reduce your sorrows, not your savings. Remind yourself that the first signs of spirituality are cheerfulness and inner peace and these characteristics should emanate from the teacher.

Spiritual books and disks are beneficial for calming the body and mind. I think that you are more likely to get restorative rest if you drift off to sleep with spiritual notions on your mind.

62... TEMPERATURE

Your brain will wake you if you are too hot or too cold. Environmental temperatures of less than 12°C (54°F) or more than 24°C (75°F) may disturb sleep. My observations are that most people sleep much better in the winter — and that most Australians use too many bed covers. Some people apparently feel more secure and comforted when they are under relatively heavy bed covers. Don't wear synthetic fabrics to bed in the summer and be aware that a healthy body generates heat so that it's okay to feel somewhat cool when you first get into bed.

Human core body temperature undergoes slight fluctuations in accordance with circadian rhythm.

Sleep laboratory studies indicate that elevated core body temperature is associated with waking during the night in the elderly.[47] Menopause aside, most of my older patients tell me that they are sure their internal temperature is higher than when they were young adults and I suspect that this is because the heat control centre in the brain is less efficient.

A deep, slow bath at a temperature of 40-41°C initially increases body temperature, but about an hour later the core body temperature drops slightly, and this drop triggers sleepiness. Many people, especially the elderly report that an evening bath helps them fall asleep more quickly and their sleep is better maintained throughout the night. Since elderly people tend to get sleepy too early in the evening, the warm bath may delay bedtime by an hour but care needs to be taken not to fall asleep in the bath! Investing in a fan or a good air conditioning system is a must for summer insomniacs.

Melatonin supplementation, taken about 2 p.m., can slightly lower core body temperature in insomniacs and give modest sleep improvements.[48] This conflicts with the common suggestion that melatonin should be taken about one hour before bedtime. Thus some trial and error is required when finding the ideal time to take melatonin.

If your feet burn in bed this could be due to –

Disorders of the nerves in the legs (neuropathy) caused by diabetes, a high sugar diet, alcohol excess, liver problems, kidney problems, thyroid dysfunction, obesity, fluid retention, nerve entrapment between third and fourth toes, vitamin B deficiencies (especially B12) or poor circulation to the feet.

Erythromelalgia is a complex nerve and circulatory condition with painful burning of the feet or hands causing the skin temperature to increase by 8°C.[49]

Recommendations for fixing burning and/or hot feet include-

•Get more physical activity.

•Rest with your feet up whenever practicable during the day.

•Avoid standing still; get a high stool to sit on for some jobs; and use a footstool when sitting.

•Massage your toes, feet and legs before bed using a good moisturizing cream (preferably an anti-inflammatory herbal cream made up by your herbalist or vitamin E cream) and then lie on the floor with your feet up for 5 — 10 minutes.

•Consult a podiatrist and get your footwear checked.

•Avoid sugar and sugary foods; if you like the taste of sweet use stevia or xylitol instead of sugar. Follow a low carbohydrate diet – see chapter 23 of my book " *Can't Lose Weight? You could have Syndrome X*"

•Improve your liver function by eating more salads, raw juicing with things such as cabbage, carrot, radish, beetroot, capsicum and citrus and take a good liver tonic

•Ensure that you have enough essential fatty acids in your diet – these are essential for healthy nerves and circulation

•Take a vitamin C supplement to improve circulation

•As a last resort try an "ice brick" on the soles of your feet in bed

Depending on the climate and the individual, you can be too cold in bed. Cold hands and feet are a common problem and may prevent or disrupt sleep. Cold exposure can cause abnormal constriction (spasm) of the blood vessels, particularly in the hands and feet (vasospastic syndrome) and this prevents the onset of sleep. Swiss researchers found that keeping the feet warm promotes a rapid onset of sleep even in normal young people.[50]

In the 'old days' people used to wear bed socks and nightcaps in winter and in some circumstances this may be helpful, particularly for those with poor circulation who live in cold climates. If you use a hot water bottle, I recommend covering these because you don't want to end up with chilblains or a burn!

Getting the temperature right obviously influences circulation and in turn this affects melatonin, blood pressure, heart rate, brain chemicals and sleep patterns. For instance, REM sleep decreases by 25 to 50 per cent in extreme arctic weather and this reduces reaction time during the day.[51]

Core body temperature is generally at its lowest at waking time and I suspect that the elderly may wake relatively early, as well as during the night, because their core temperatures may fluctuate more than younger people. Those with an underactive thyroid gland will have an abnormally low body core temperature that will usually interfere with sleep. Take your temperature before you get out of bed in the morning, while you are still totally relaxed and still; if its lower than 36 degrees centigrade, your blood tests will probably confirm an underactive thyroid gland.

63... THOUGHTS

Insomniacs commonly say that their thoughts continuously whirl around their brain or that the same thought recurs repetitively when they *try* to sleep. Humans are thinking creatures so it's useless telling people not to think. However, you can stop endlessly talking about your worries and never talk about insomnia except with your practitioner. Every time you think and talk about something this gets embedded in your brain.

A solution for *some* people may be to *try* to keep awake, because insomniacs seem to fall asleep very quickly when they are out. During yoga relaxation, students are supposed to become relaxed but alert; however, I've noticed that professed insomniacs often fall asleep within a few minutes. There's a psychological experiment known as the 'polar bear test'. If someone tells you *not* to think about a polar bear you invariably visualize a large white bear. If someone tells you to relax, do you relax or does this advice irritate you? If you are told *not* to worry, does this alleviate worries? If you are asked to sit quietly for five minutes and concentrate on your main problem, other things may pop into your mind. Psychologists called this 'ironic processing'.

For some people it might be a relief to feel free to focus on their problems but for most insomniacs it is better to divert unwanted thoughts. Perhaps have a specific worry time during the day, think about what you can do about your problems, how you can offset them, or get help for these problems or your attitudes about them. You might write down the issues that concern you, and put this list in a drawer so that the issues are symbolically and literally out of sight. You can get the get the list out at any time *except* at night.

We all have worries and some have more than their share. Assigning blame, replaying the problems over and over in our minds, feeling that we are unfairly treated, and constantly repeating our injuries to others not only imposes a strain on relationships and friendships, but puts more 'troubling' imprints on your brain. Even relatively small problems can become magnified and cause sleeping problems.

If you are not prepared to do something about a particular problem — or get help — you should somehow find a way of living with it so that you can enjoy your life. You have a mind so you can examine your thoughts, speech, behavior and motives, and you can plan improvement — but, not in bed.

In my yoga classes, I sometimes get the students to sit quietly for ten minutes and focus on whatever thoughts come into their heads. Afterwards, some of them tell me that they couldn't think of a thing! The human brain can be very perverse and I am not sure that anyone knows where thoughts really come from. You may not be entirely responsible for everything that comes into your head and, if you believe that there are noble thoughts floating around, there may be mischievous thoughts, so you need to use your discrimination.

Do not *try* to suppress your thoughts at night but redirect them. As soon as an unwanted thought pops into your head tell yourself you'll think about that tomorrow but now you have another plan. You might listen to an audio tape, silently repeat a verse thinking of the words and meaning, or visualize your imaginary country cottage retreat, or picture your ideal resting place — perhaps near a gentle stream in a rain forest, or by the sea or in the mountains. This is called 'imagery distraction' and it can reduce the time it takes to get to sleep.[52] I have given an example of a diversionary technique in Appendix III.

Simple breathing techniques tend not to work because they don't occupy enough of your mind to block out worries. The right side of your brain is mainly the creative side whilst the left is more practical or rational, so you may need a combination technique such as visualizing while repeating words.

- Train yourself to be a positive thinker. The best system is to be aware of your thoughts (and speech) and ask yourself if you've developed the habit of negative thinking. As a great sage once said: *'Your worst enemy cannot harm you as much as your own unguarded thoughts.'*

- Avoid *thinking about sleep* after dinner. You'll need to think about it a little during the day so that you can plan your strategies.

- Sleep is instinctive and it doesn't require your thinking processes, except to work out strategies *before bed* that will allow your body to recuperate at night and let your brain do its nighttime sorting, learning and resting.

Of course, you can't pretend that problems and suffering don't exist or avoid dealing with them, and you need to use your judgement about the amount of time you spend sorting through your worries during daytime. If you don't consciously work on your problems, they will pop into your mind anyway and this is more likely to occur when you are lying in bed.

64... TINNITUS

Ringing, buzzing, and other abnormal noises in the ears may be accompanied by hearing loss and dizziness, and these symptoms cause anxiety and prevent sleep. Firstly, get a medical check from an ear nose and throat specialist because there are different causes of tinnitus, including impacted ear wax, ear infections, a nutrient deficiency and high blood pressure or nerve damage.

Medical trials have shown the following results:

In clinical trials hypnosis gave some benefit to 68 per cent of cases[53] and biofeedback gave a 50 per cent improvement, compared to 30 per cent for acupuncture and 10 per cent for cinnarizine (an antihistamine).[54] A study of army personnel with occupational noise exposure found that low levels of vitamin B12 were significantly more prevalent among those with tinnitus — and injections of that vitamin provided some relief.[55]

Natural supplements to improve the circulation of blood to the inner ear can help to reduce tinnitus and dizziness. These include circulatory herbs such as ginkgo, bilberry, hawthorn, rosehip, ginger, garlic, turmeric and chilli, and vitamin C.

Specific nutrient supplements of minerals can help such as magnesium, calcium, zinc, manganese, boron and selenium. These minerals are needed to keep the inner ear structures healthy and strong and I have found that they can really make a big difference in reducing tinnitus and dizziness due to inflammatory and/or degenerative changes in the inner ear.

Vitamin D deficiency can manifest as dizziness and tinnitus and if you do not get enough exposure to sunlight I would recommend a blood test to measure your levels of vitamin D. You may need to take between 400 to 1000 I.U daily of vitamin D to get relief. Good food sources of vitamin D are sardines and organic eggs (make sure that you eat the yolks).

You could also try ear drops using a small dropper bottle that you can buy from a pharmacy: Put 20 ml of either glycerine or sesame oil into the bottle. Add six drops of lavender and six drops of rose oil. Shake before use. Put 2 – 3 drops of the mix into each ear once or twice daily, having one of the doses before bed.

> Caution: Do not put the dropper itself into the ear because you may damage the eardrum. Tilt your head to one side, put the dropper near the external opening of the ear and you will feel the remedy go in.

Try using a soft pillow because the ears are very sensitive to hard pressure and it's worth spending around $130 for a pure down pillow.

Tinnitus is difficult to treat and most therapies require some months' treatment so patience is needed.

Sound therapy can also help. As a diversion from tinnitus, you can use music that you enjoy, or 'talking' books that are available in libraries and bookstores. The Australian Tinnitus Association Ltd sells noise generators and relaxing music and you can get more information at http://www.tinnitus.asn.au/tinnitus.htm or phone 02 8382 3333, or write to PO Box 660, Woollahra, NSW 1350.

65... TRAUMA AND GRIEF

Traumatic experiences and grief obviously affect sleep. Depending on the circumstances, it can be necessary to take an antidepressant drug or sleeping pills. For more information on these medications see Appendix IV.

I am not giving simplistic advice about traumatic events but everything seems worse when you are inside and alone, so getting outdoors, and having company will help sustain you. Continuously talking about the problem or dreaming about it may or may not be releasing (cathartic), and in some people it may make matters worse, especially if you get inappropriate feedback or advice that conflicts with your wishes. There is an association that can provide links to support groups and counsellors:

National Association for Loss & Grief,
PO Box 214, Essendon VIC 3040 Australia
Phone 03 9351 0358 or visit http://www.nalagvic.org.au

66... WINDING DOWN REQUIREMENTS

If you are overstimulated, trying to relax is like trying to put a car in reverse when travelling at speed. The overstimulation may be from work, conflict, exercise or an outing. Entertainers in particular often need a long winding down time because when they are on stage their adrenal glands get very activated. That's when television may be helpful, whereas a standard relaxing tape may be irritating. Another option is to go outside and look at the stars or have a leisurely walk.

Ideally poor sleepers need a long, steady winding down before bed and at least brief relaxation periods throughout the day to avoid a build-up of tension. When you have a tea or coffee break, be mindful of enjoying the drink. Get away from your desk and go outside for at least a short time during your lunch break. If you have children play some outdoors games with them or take them for a walk. Herbal sedative remedies may be helpful and these are covered in Chapter 4.

67... WITHDRAWAL SYMPTOMS

When you stop taking various drugs and compounds, you may suffer from withdrawal symptoms, including insomnia. Withdrawal effects may occur when you stop alcohol, caffeine, nicotine and various social and pharmaceutical drugs. There is no evidence that herbal sedatives cause such withdrawal effects but it is possible if high doses are taken long-term.

Although many pharmaceuticals prescribed for the nervous system are not technically classified as addictive, they may lead to tolerance (higher doses are required to get an effect) or dependency. If you gradually reduce your intake, with the supervision of your doctor, this usually prevents withdrawal symptoms. Withdrawal symptoms can also be reduced by taking magnesium and vitamin C supplements.

68.. WORRY ABOUT SLEEP

This is technically referred to as conditioned insomnia. In some cases, the thought or desire to sleep and the act of getting ready for bed, triggers anxiety and the inability to sleep. That's why I suggest that poor sleepers avoid talking and thinking about sleep, especially in the evening. And, get everything and yourself ready for bed *early* in the evening so that when a 'sleepiness wave' arrives you can go calmly to bed, as outlined above under 'sleep routine'.

Every thought and word gets imprinted on the brain, and your brain automatically registers insomnia thoughts and words. Some people tell their friends how they can never get to sleep and they receive very little sympathy because it's boring conversation and because the insomniac might fall asleep very readily during a concert or at a restaurant — when *not thinking about or wishing to sleep*.

During relaxation therapy (that doesn't mention the word 'relax' or 'sleep') I may tell patients that they have to focus on every word I say and remain alert; and the insomniacs often fall asleep within a few minutes!

In conclusion

Restorative sleep is health enhancing and anti ageing and you should take some steps to get your quota of this deeply healing and economical remedy. Insomniacs need to focus on enjoying their lives and improving their health with holistic strategies, and not get too obsessed about their sleep.

Chapter 4

RELAXING AND ANTISTRESS HERBS

Relaxant herbs do *not* overcome some of the factors that cause poor sleep. For instance, if your nutrient intake is inadequate or you are anaemic, relaxant herbs will not offset dietary deficiencies or anaemia. In other words, you may need to establish the cause of your insomnia rather than taking a remedy.

Most professional herbalists use formulas that are much stronger than over-the-counter natural remedies and their formulas are designed to treat the whole person. My twenty-five years' experience is that the side effects of medicinal herbs are minimal and many insomniacs can be treated more effectively if they have some herbal help to calm them down at night.

Herbs have varying strengths depending on soil, climate, stage of growth and so on, and natural variations are not necessarily a reflection on manufacturing quality. Some herbs, such as St John's wort, have known specific therapeutic compounds and products may be modified to ensure given levels of particular constituents. However, all plants contain many hundreds of compounds and they produce a wide range of effects that are often subtle and indirect. Many herbs help the digestion, because of their aromatic oil content or bitter compounds, and that is one of the reasons why insomnia remedies may be more effective if half the dose is taken after dinner and half before bed.

The following are some of the herbs that are helpful for insomnia:

HOPS (HUMULUS LUPULUS)

In traditional herbal medicine, hops is used to relax the body and mind and to relieve insomnia. I organized tests for phytestrogenic activity and the assays showed this herb to have a higher level than that of any other plant. However, the dosage of herbs is around one teaspoon daily so if you want a phytestrogenic effect for menopausal insomnia, I suggest eating *foods* such as whole ground flaxseeds, sprouts and soy.

Scientific studies in animals indicate that herbal hops not only has sedative and sleep-inducing properties but it is hypothermic (cooling), anticonvulsant and somewhat analgesic.

In Germany, where doctors are trained in herbal medicine, the official herbal guide lists hops for mood disturbances such as restlessness, as well as anxiety and sleep disturbances.[1]

I prescribe hops as a liquid extract, for evening use only, usually one dose after dinner and one dose before bed, the maximum dose being 2.5 ml daily.

Hops herbal pillows and baths are traditional sleep remedies but the aroma is somewhat unpleasant so I suggest adding lavender to any external treatment.

Caution: Hops is not generally prescribed for depressed people.

ZIZIPHUS (ZIZYPHUS) – THE CHINESE SLEEP HERB

Ziziphus spinosa is a Traditional Chinese Herbal Medicine that is being used with increasing frequency by Western Herbalists. It has been described in many Chinese herbal texts as being useful in nourishing the heart and calming the spirit[2], and is still being employed today for the same reasons. Ziziphus' actions are much more specific and less far reaching than most other well known herbal medicines. It is useful as a sedative and is able to relieve the symptoms of anxiety and has also been found to reduce elevated blood pressure. As a result of these refined actions, it is indicated in conditions such as insomnia due to nervous exhaustion, anxiety, palpitations, hypertension and night sweats. It has also been noted to be valuable in anorexia, nervous exhaustion, forgetfulness and nightmares[3]. It is employed by some herbalists for insomnia caused by excessive sweating, such as that experienced in menopausal insomnia and feverish conditions causing difficulty falling asleep.[4]

Much of the scientific data that confirms Ziziphus' efficacy and safety is written in Mandarin. However, most Western herbalists who use Ziziphus with some regularity, state that its increased popularity in western herbal medicine has been an invaluable addition to their herbal dispensary for use in patients who experience insomnia.

The use of Ziziphus by traditional Chinese herbalists is cautioned in patients with severe diarrhoea[5]. There are no other reported warnings or precautions associated with the use of this herb.

This information has been provided by naturopath Simone Abaron who works in Dr. Cabot's Broadway Holistic Health Centre in Sydney.

PASSION FLOWER (PASSIFLORA INCARNATA)

This is the wild version of the vine that we grow for its edible fruits. Passion flower herb has a long history of use for various nervous complaints. Its sedative and antianxiety effects make it useful for insomnia, palpitations, muscle spasms and stress. You will find passion flower in many over-the-counter formulas for insomnia and anxiety.

A clinical trial indicates that passion flower is just as effective as oxazepam (a sedative pharmaceutical) for general anxiety and the herb has a lower incidence of performance impairment compared to the pharmaceutical.[6] The tranquilizing effects of passion flower have been confirmed in at least three trials and it may be a useful adjunct in the treatment of opiate withdrawal — with practitioner monitoring. The specific combination of valerian and passion flower is often helpful for insomnia.

KAVA (PIPER METHYTHISTICUM)

My experience is that most cases of insomnia are linked to anxiety and I consider that kava is an effective natural antianxiety medicine. Professional herbalists prescribe kava for anxiety, restlessness, insomnia, muscle tension, stress headaches, and bladder and gastric problems linked to nervousness. Studies indicate that kava may help reduce withdrawal symptoms of pharmaceutical sedatives.[7]

The main advantage of kava is that it lowers anxiety in the majority of cases within a week and does not impair learning or reaction time.[8] In fact one trial showed that it improves reaction time and word recognition performance.[9] Kava also reduces anxiety and enhances wellbeing in menopausal women.[10] and is equivalent to some sedative drugs in measurements of anxiety, aggression and tension.[11] A systematic review of the evidence indicates that kava extract is a herbal treatment option for anxiety that is worthy of consideration.[12]

The medicinal form of kava is not the same as the alcoholic drink, although the traditional drinking of kava is not a problem unless it is excessive. In the Pacific Islands, kava beverage has been an important part of ceremonies for many centuries, primarily to promote 'togetherness'. The drink is said to produce feelings of contentment, fluent and lively speech, muscle relaxation and deep, restful sleep without a hangover. If you chew the root it produces a spicy, bitter taste that develops into a peppery sensation and the tongue may become numb. In traditional medicine, kava in various forms is also used to treat a wide range of conditions including headaches, urinary problems, inflammation, joint problems and topically for skin conditions.

A six-week trial showed that kava was effective for treating stress-induced insomnia.[13] Kava combined with valerian is also helpful although in one trial there were a few reported side effects including vivid dreams, gastric discomfort and dizziness.

Caution: There have been cases of severe liver toxicity reported but these have involved products such as standardised acetone extracts and very high doses (neither of which are used in Australia), or the patients had existing liver problems or they were taking other products some of which were not identified. In one case of purported kava toxicity, for example, a woman developed hepatitis while taking kava but she had been on an alcohol binge and treated herself with paracetamol. There are many causes of hepatitis; a major alcohol binge can damage the liver and even common over-the-counter painkillers such as paracetamol have the warning 'administer with care in patients with hepatic dysfunction'.

To my knowledge, only one case of kava toxicity has been reported in Australia and according to published reports, the person was also taking an unidentified compound. Nevertheless, it is possible that some individuals may be peculiarly sensitive to kava — or to any particular food or plant.

Current Australian regulations for Kava

Products to be made of the dried root or water extracts of the dried root.

- The daily dose should not exceed 250 mg of kavalactone components, or 125 mg in each tablet or capsule, or the rhizome does not exceed 3 g in a tea bag.[14]

- To be prescribed by practitioners so that patients may be monitored for adverse reactions. Contact the prescribing practitioner if you have an unexpected illness while taking kava (or any remedy) or if you develop loss of appetite, swelling of the abdomen, yellowing of the skin or eyes, dark urine or other unusual symptoms.

- Do not take kava for more than two months without a break, otherwise use at irregular intervals. A liver function test is recommended every two months if taken long-term.

Those who should not take kava:

- People with liver diseases or suspected liver problems.

- Pregnant women and children under twelve years.

•Anyone consuming more than two alcoholic drinks per day.

•Anyone taking any social or pharmaceutical drug that may affect the liver.

•Epileptics and those with Parkinson's disease.

VALERIAN (VALERIANA OFFICINALIS)

Valerian is the most commonly prescribed insomnia herb. It is routinely prescribed by medical practitioners in Germany for restlessness and sleeping disorders linked to nervous conditions.[15] A number of medical trials show that valerian has positive effects on sleep structure and self-perception of sleep quality without causing significant adverse effects. One group of researchers reported that their study showed an extremely low number of adverse effects during the valerian treatment periods (3 side effects compared to 18 on placebo).[16] Another study showed that valerian was just as effective as oxazepam (Serepax).

Valerian can be useful for other problems including anxiety, hyperactivity, headaches, and spasms such as colic and menstrual cramps.

Laboratory studies indicate that valerian contains the sleep hormone melatonin but whether the medicinal dose of the herb provides a therapeutic quantity of melatonin is debatable, however, it is possible that only a tiny amount is needed to 'top up' the body's own production of this hormone.

Different species of valerian have been used in Asia, the Middle East and Mexico and a common feature of all the species is that they are also helpful for digestive problems.

Mexican Valerian

Mexican valerian (*Valeriana mexicana* or *Valeriana edulis*) is similar therapeutically and has similar compounds compared with the more widely used European valerian. A polysomnogram study compared the two valerians and found that both herbs increased

REM sleep, increased sleep efficiency and decreased morning fatigue but European valerian was more effective in these areas. However, Mexican valerian was more effective at increasing stage three and four deep sleep, reducing stage one and two light sleep, and decreasing waking episodes.[17]

> Caution: My experience is that a small percentage of patients react unfavorably to valerian; some report that it makes them somewhat sleepy the morning after and a few patients say it makes them 'jittery'. These effects have not been reported in trials and may reflect individual sensitivity or idiosyncratic reactions. However, a study on rats indicates that valerian acts on GABA receptors in the brain and therefore this herb may not be appropriate for everyone and it would be unwise to take it before surgery.

Although the taste 'grows on you' I recommend tablets for first-time users rather than teas or extracts and suggest taking half the dose before or after dinner, and half the dose before bed.

A woman attempted suicide by taking 20 times the label dose of valerian. After 30 minutes, she complained of fatigue, abdominal cramping, chest tightness, light-headedness and feet and hand tremor. Her pupils dilated and she had a fine hand tremor but all other tests were normal.[18] This demonstrates that valerian is relatively benign and also supports my contention that common medicinal herbs are unlikely to cause fatalities but overdoses can make you very ill.

There have been some unfavorable papers on valerian in medical journals, but these have not stood up to scrutiny.

LEMON BALM (MELISSA OFFICINALIS)

A German medical study of 68 insomnia patients showed that a combination of lemon balm and valerian improved sleep quality and had a positive effect on daily wellbeing and anxiety compared to placebo. There were no 'hangover' or rebound effects and only three adverse effects were linked to the herbs (headache, stomach ache and cramps), however, it is not clear whether these side effects were actually caused by the herbs.[19] Other studies have confirmed that this combination is well tolerated and appears to improve sleep quality.

Lemon balm is also used for treating irritable bowel, flatulence, dyspepsia, restlessness and daytime nervousness. For irritable bowel symptoms, lemon balm combines well with herbal peppermint.

ST JOHN'S WORT (HYPERICUM PERFORATUM)

Traditional therapeutic uses of St John's wort include nerve pain, anxiety, headaches, and infections. It has a long history of use for soothing injuries and as an external healing agent.

At least 15 medical studies have shown that St John's wort herb is more helpful than placebo for treating *mild to moderate depression*. I find this remarkable considering that many medical studies use much lower doses of this herb than professional herbalists. There is a strong link between insomnia and depression and I prescribe St John's wort for both problems either separately in tablet form or as a liquid extract in a formula. There is also an excellent product available which combines St Johns wort with B group vitamins, magnesium and other minerals to balance the nervous system. For more information ring the Health Advisory Service on 02 4655 8855 in Australia and 623 344 3232 in USA.

Caution: There are reported adverse reactions but these are about ten times less than with pharmaceutical antidepressants. I have never had a problem with St John's wort in my clinic although some patients do not want to take it because they have read something adverse. For example, a USA study showing St John's wort to be non-effective for treating severe depression was widely publicized, however, the same study also showed that Zoloft (a pharmaceutical with a sales figures of over US$2 billion) was equally ineffective.[20] The daily dose of St John's wort in the trial was between 900 mg to 1500 mg.

If medical researchers are going to 'test' herbal medicine, perhaps they should employ a herbalist to get the dose and the indications correct. Using a guaranteed potency remedy I might prescribe a daily tablet dose of up to 5,000 mg or liquid extract of 6,000 ml daily and I would recommend dietary and lifestyle changes as well — and more importantly I would *not* prescribe it for *major* depression.

CHAMOMILE (CHAMOMILLA RECUTITA)

Chamomile has a long history of use in Europe as a mild sedative, and is often taken as a tea before bed, although I suggest half a cup only for older people because all fluid is somewhat diuretic. Most herbalists prescribe German chamomile and the *flower* is used to make teas, tablets and concentrated extracts.

In Germany chamomile is currently officially used as an internal remedy for gastrointestinal spasms and inflammatory diseases of the gastrointestinal tract.[21]

The usual dose is 3 g of the herb three or four times daily, made as a tea, covered for 5-10 minutes, then strained. If you don't like the taste of chamomile, you can make the tea from ginger water. To make the ginger water, simmer finely chopped ginger root in water for about five minutes. Use half to two teaspoons of ginger per cup of water, depending on your taste. You can sweeten with honey or stevia.

Chamomile is recommended as a bath for inflammation and irritation of the skin, and as a mouthwash or gargle for inflamed mouth and throat. Gargles should always be tepid, so that the remedy feels neither hot nor cold. A hot tea can also be used as an inhalation to soothe the respiratory system and help clear the nasal passages. I mention these other uses because seemingly unrelated problems may disturb sleep.

An old study showed that chamomile tea (two teabags) induced deep sleep in 10 out of 12 patients undergoing heart catheterization even though the procedure commonly causes pain and anxiety.[22] The tea did not cause any adverse effects on the heart.

Chamomile *oil* comes in different qualities, the most potent being a deep blue oil. It has an interesting apple-like odor and you need only one drop used as a perfume to provide a sedating effect. A scientific study showed that inhaled chamomile oil is sedative and improves mood compared to placebo.[23] The oil is not used internally and other ways of using aromatic oils are given under the heading 'aromatherapy' in Chapter 5.

You can see from this brief overview that chamomile is ideal for people with digestive irritation coupled with anxiety, both of which are linked to insomnia.

> Caution: Chamomile is in the daisy family (Asteraceae) and some plants in this family are allergens, especially in people with eczema and asthma. Most authoritative texts and monographs state that side effects are extremely rare. There are many thousands of plants in this family and you should never pick and consume any plant that you cannot positively identify. For some herbs 'we' use the total plant while for other we use only a specific portion, such as the root or leaves; or flowers in the case of chamomile. If you self-treat you need to know this information for each plant.

NOTE: Tradition and scientific evidence indicate that insomnia herbs need at least a few weeks' treatment to improve sleep. In most of the medical trials of herbs, the dosages are well below that which most Australian professional herbalists would prescribe but you must follow the label doses of remedies because the strengths can vary.

When you obtain a herbal formula from a herbalist, insist on getting a list of all the ingredients. If there is not enough room on the label to write everything in a formula, ask for it to be written separately. In principle, you should know *everything* you are taking because you may want to get a repeat of the same remedy or you may have an allergic reaction and want to avoid this in the future. With sensitive people I often give small 'test' bottles of individual herbs before making up a formula. If patients need herbal remedies for a long period of time, I often alternate a formula because this avoids potential toxicity problems and possible adaptation (that is, the body may get used to a remedy and then it doesn't work any more).

- There are varying strengths of herbs and medications, and you must take the label dose of any remedy.

- If you are on other medications, you need to discuss additional remedies with your practitioner.

- It is obviously risky to combine sedative herbs with pharmaceuticals prescribed for the nervous system because they may augment or mar the desired therapeutic effect.

- Some of my patients say that sedative herbs make them feel 'groggy' in the morning. If this happens, I suggest that they be taken in one dose before dinner or use a lower dose — or try something else.

Chapter 5

SUPPLEMENTS AND OTHER NATURAL THERAPIES

B VITAMINS

The B group vitamins in general are required for nerve structure and functioning, and the nervous system is involved in various aspects of sleep. A varied diet with foods in as natural a state as possible should supply you with all the essential nutrients. Biotin deficiency is linked to many conditions such as dry skin, red painful tongue, dry eyes, fatigue and insomnia. Niacinamide and inositol supplementation is helpful for some insomniacs.

Vitamin B12 is necessary for the structure and function of nerve fibres and cells, and it also influences melatonin. A deficiency of this vitamin causes anaemia and a wide range of potentially severe physical and mental problems. My experience is that many elderly people in particular have improvements in general wellbeing when they are given a form of vitamin B12 that they can absorb, such as injections. Six weekly injections of vitamin B 12 are much preferred to tablets if you have digestive or intestinal problems or are over 60 years of age. It is easy to check your levels of vitamin B 12 with a simple blood test. Methylcobalamin, a particular form of vitamin B12, is considered useful for treating circadian rhythm problems in patients with central nervous system disorders and blindness.[1] These problems are linked to insomnia.

ESSENTIAL FATTY ACIDS

Essential fatty acids are necessary for the structure of membranes around cells and other body tissues. Researchers suggest that essential fatty acids have beneficial effects on nerve membranes[2] including the receiving and transmitting of information. Foods that contain vital essential fatty acids include fish, nuts, seeds (especially flaxseeds), whole grains, avocado and olive oil.

For more information on healthy dietary fats and the brain see page 52

Fish oil supplementation is a concentrated source of essential fatty acids and is very helpful for a number of nerve-related disorders. I usually prescribe it combined with an antioxidant such as vitamin E. Fish oil is suggested as a sleep supplement because it helps brain cells, it is anti-inflammatory and has various health benefits indirectly linked to sleep — such as relieving joint and circulatory problems.

MAGNESIUM

Magnesium is recommended for many physical and emotional disorders, and supplementation helps many of these disorders. When we are stressed, our bodies use up our magnesium stores quickly. Foods rich in magnesium include seaweeds, whole grains, nuts, soy and molasses. Molasses is a good tonic but may be contaminated with pesticides so make sure you buy organic brands.

One study showed that magnesium supplementation improves sleep quality by increasing slow wave sleep and decreasing adrenal stress hormones.[3]

Magnesium supplementation can be dramatically effective for muscle cramps and spasms, leg pains and restless legs. I have found that magnesium supplementation is a must in those with anxiety, panic attacks, high blood pressure, heart palpitations and migraine headaches.

Poor sleep apparently reduces magnesium levels in your cells, which means that you are less able to exercise. Supplementation of 100 to 400 mg of magnesium daily usually improves sleep and your capacity to exercise. Some people may benefit by taking more than 400mg daily, and although magnesium is generally safe you should be guided by your practitioner. Excess magnesium can cause diarrhoea.

I call magnesium the "great relaxer" as it helps to balance the whole nervous system in a desirable way and thus not only helps with stress induced insomnia but many other nervous and cardiovascular complaints.

MELATONIN

Melatonin is a sleep-promoting hormone produced naturally in the body from the amino acid tryptophan. In most people, natural melatonin secretion starts about 9 p.m. to 10 p.m. Melatonin is made by the pineal gland, which is located in the back part of the mid-brain.

Some trials using melatonin supplementation may not have produced appropriate results because of the timing and dosage. Currently there is no general agreement on dosages and these may need to be varied according to age, body weight, general health and the type of sleep problem.

Melatonin therapy helps some people with REM sleep behavior disorders related to neurologic conditions.[4] Patients were prescribed between 3mg to 12 mg and some side effects were noted including headaches, morning sleepiness and delusions/ hallucinations — which were reversed when the doses were lowered.

A study of elderly insomniacs showed that a dosage of only 0.3 mg taken 30 minutes before bed was the most effective dosage, while a 3 mg dose caused a reduction of body temperature.[5] A number of studies confirm that melatonin is especially helpful for elderly insomniacs but the dose may need to be quite low initially — to avoid adverse reactions.

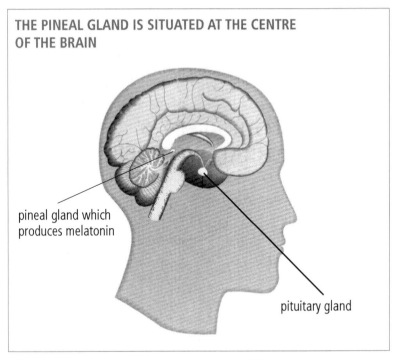

THE PINEAL GLAND IS SITUATED AT THE CENTRE OF THE BRAIN

pineal gland which produces melatonin

pituitary gland

Melatonin may help some people come off benzodiazepine sleeping pills.[6] The withdrawal from these sleeping pills is not always possible in very long term users, and it needs to be done very slowly and requires monitoring by a medical practitioner.

About 77 per cent of blind people with no perception of light may have abnormal circadian rhythms and sleep problems, while those with light perception sleep better.[7] When totally blind people were given 5 mg melatonin one hour before bedtime this gave them increased total sleep time and sleep efficiency.[8]

Melatonin is an antioxidant and free radical scavenger.[9] It protects healthy cells from toxicity caused by cancer radiation and chemotherapy treatment.[10] It interacts with growth and adrenal hormones, and may reduce oestrogen levels. Theoretically, melatonin may help prevent and treat some types of cancer. However, this is still very controversial and be aware that it has not been fully evaluated.

Caution: If you want natural hormones (such as melatonin) in Australia, I suggest you find a compounding pharmacist in your locality to obtain a list of doctors who are prepared to prescribe them. In Australia you need a doctor's script to get **real** melatonin. Homoeopathic melatonin is very weak and cannot be compared to therapeutic doses of melatonin.

Although you may be able to obtain hormones on the Internet *do not self-treat*. You don't know how these products are manufactured, and the promotional material is invariably an exaggeration of the benefits or a misrepresentation of the science. Furthermore, four out of six melatonin supplements in the USA were found to contain unidentified impurities.[11]

The research on melatonin is complicated and until the evidence is clarified, do not take melatonin if you have epilepsy, or if you are on warfarin and anticoagulant pharmaceuticals. Large doses of melatonin, may lead to hypothermia (low body heat), and cause a release of prolactin that will diminish male libido.

When six children with neurological defects were given melatonin for their sleep complaints four of them had *seizure increases or new seizure activity*.[12] One U.S. government report indicates that long-term use of melatonin can build up in the body and may create new problems.[13]

TRYPTOPHAN

L-tryptophan is an essential amino acid present in foods, notably meat, poultry, eggs, dairy products, and some nuts and seeds — notably pumpkin seeds, cashews and sesame seeds. You must get tryptophan from your food because your body cannot manufacture it. This amino acid is involved in niacin metabolism and can be converted to other compounds in the body including 5-hydroxytryptophan and serotonin (chemical name 5-hydroxytryptamine). Serotonin is commonly described as a mood-enhancing neurotransmitter and it helps regulate sleep, appetite and body temperature. We know that serotonin helps reduce depression because some antidepressant pharmaceuticals conserve serotonin in the brain. Tryptophan may also help some cases of depression.

Indirectly, tryptophan increases production of the sleep hormone melatonin, and it is known that low levels of tryptophan are linked to decreased production of melatonin by the body.[14]

Dietary tryptophan may be converted to serotonin but in order to make this conversion your body needs other nutrients – namely Vitamin B 6 (pyridoxine), folic acid, vitamin C, and magnesium. Nothing in your body works in isolation. L-tryptophan does not get absorbed as such into the brain (via the blood brain barrier) but its converted form, 5-hydroxytryptophan, does get into the brain.

I want to reduce your fears about tryptophan. It is true that many years ago a particular tryptophan product caused a serious, painful muscle and joint disorder (eosinophilic-myalgia syndrome) that resulted in the death of 37 people in the USA. However, the tryptophan that caused the problem was a particular Japanese product that utilized genetically engineered bacteria to produce the tryptophan. Nevertheless, most governments throughout the world either banned tryptophan or markedly reduced the dosages that could be sold without a doctor's script. This is the equivalent of banning vegetables because one supplier used excess pesticides. The end result is that the Australian Government actually approves and gives licences to over-the-counter products that contain less than a therapeutic dose. Medical Practitioners can obtain stronger products from suppliers and compounding pharmacists.

Tryptophan supplementation does not work for all insomniacs, but it can work well for others with sleeping problems and depression. A study indicated that those who reported waking up between three and six times throughout the night all improved, whereas other categories of insomniacs did not.[15] You will need to experiment with your own doctor and a compounding pharmacist to get the larger doses that may be needed.

Caution: Tryptophan supplementation is not recommended during pregnancy and lactation, or for people with asthma and lupus. It should not be taken with some pharmaceuticals including antidepressants, pain medications, anti-anxiety drugs and carbidopa.

ACUPUNCTURE

A German trial in a sleep laboratory showed that acupuncture is helpful for relieving insomnia, although the researchers did not rule out the influence of the therapist. (I can't see that it matters if the personality or the 'vibes' of a practitioner contribute to better health. It is likely that this happens with many holistic doctors and natural therapists because these practitioners spend a relatively long time with each patient.)

A number of Chinese reports support acupuncture as an effective therapy for some nerve-related problems, and sites in the nervous system where acupuncture signals are integrated are also involved in sleep-wake cycles.[16]

ACUPRESSURE

There are two acupressure points that may help balance the energies in your body and promote restful sleep. They are called the "Spirit Gate" and the "Inner Gate".

Turn the palms of your hands upwards.

- The Spirit Gate is located just below the prominent wrist crease and in line with the little finger (that is, towards the fingers). You'll feel a slight indentation in the area.
- The Inner Gate is located 2½ finger widths up from the wrist crease and in line with the ring finger.

For the Spirit Gate I suggest using the thumb, in line with the wrist crease and pressing down. For the Inner Gate use the tops of two fingers vertically, in line with the tendons. The aim is to apply steady (not extreme) pressure on each hand for one minute — which is about six rounds of calm breathing.

LEFT HAND - PALM UP

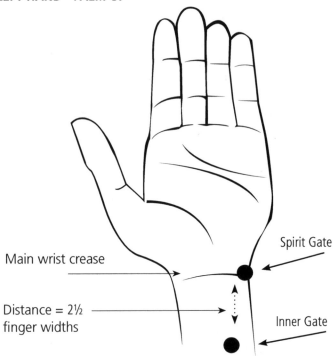

Main wrist crease

Distance = 2½
finger widths

Spirit Gate

Inner Gate

RIGHT HAND - PALM UP

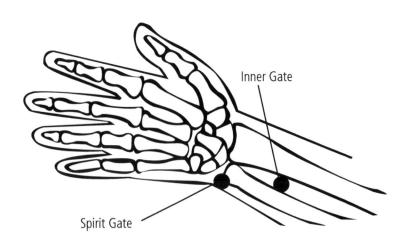

Inner Gate

Spirit Gate

AROMATHERAPY

Aromatherapy is the use of aromatic plant oils for therapeutic purposes, and when used appropriately it is safe, effective and economical. The oils are either inhaled or placed on the skin. These types of oils are absorbed into the body through the breath or through the skin and then excreted via the breath, faeces and urine. The absorption time is between 5 — 90 minutes and excretion via urine is variable, probably averaging about four hours.

Three scientific trials confirm that aromatherapy has a significant, beneficial effect on agitation compared to placebo.[17] Agitation is obviously linked to insomnia.

For the purposes of insomnia and relaxation, the aroma does not have to be powerful and the following are general guidelines:

• About six drops of oil in a whole body bath or footbath.

• One drop as a perfume — you need only a 'whiff'.

• Three to six drops on a tissue under the pillow. Aromatic oils may be more effective if inhaled steadily throughout the night in this way, especially for insomniacs who wake during the night.

• About three to six drops massaged into the scalp

• 10—20 drops in 50 g aqueous cream or in 50 ml almond oil for an external foot or body massage. This quantity will last for a number of treatments.

Lavender oil

Some medical trials confirm that lavender oil can be helpful for restlessness and sleeping problems. One report maintains that it is just as effective as pharmaceutical sleeping pills or tranquillizers.[18] Some patients with abdominal problems such as bloating and irritable bowel syndrome, say that a gentle abdominal massage with lavender oil helps alleviate nighttime intestinal discomfort. A lavender oil massage also helps some cases of muscle pain and sore feet, and scientists have confirmed that this oil has some pain reducing activity when used externally.[19]

Lavender oil contains perillyl alcohol, which is currently being studied for its anti-cancer effects, and it may be useful to add a little to skin lotions, not only to alleviate stress but possibly to help prevent skin cancer. In addition, lavender as a perfume may help you handle stress more effectively during the day, and therefore help insomnia by preventing a build up of tension by the evening. Lavender oil has anti-inflammatory activity and I find it helpful for insect bites and irritated skin. On an insect bite I would apply one drop undiluted but for large areas use it diluted as indicated above.

Anything that is physically soothing is likely to benefit sleep. Lavender pillows and toys are available, and having a faint whiff of lavender over a long period is known to reduce unintentional muscle movement.

> Caution: Some herbalists use lavender flowers as an internal herbal remedy, the dose being about a teaspoon once or twice daily for stomach, intestinal and gallbladder complaints. However, the oil is not used internally. Don't confuse the herb with the oil because the oil represents about two per cent of the plant's contents and aromatic oils are surprisingly potent.

All aromatic oils are concentrated products but in 25 years of using lavender oil I have only had one patient experience an allergic reaction.

Cedarwood oil

Cedarwood oil contains cedrol and when this is inhaled it has marked sedative effects.[20] Some people find that cedarwood oil is also helpful for hair loss when massaged into the scalp, and given that hair loss may be linked to stress this may be worth trying. In addition, when you are stressed there is usually tension in the scalp, and simply massaging the scalp may help you relax at night. I suggest about 6 drops of cedarwood oil as a scalp massage.

Other sedative aromatic oils are basil, chamomile, marjoram, and melissa (lemon balm).

> Caution: Sensitive people may be allergic to aromatic oils, so I recommend testing one drop of oil on the inside of the elbow before using on the scalp or body. Do not use any aromatic oil internally unless specifically prescribed by a qualified practitioner.

BATHS

Fourteen female insomniacs had baths at around 40°C, 1½ to 2 hours before bedtime, and this increased body temperature early in the evening and improved slow wave sleep in the early part of the sleep period and improved sleep continuity.[21] A number of studies have confirmed that hot baths before bed improve sleep quality in both young and old people, whereas cool baths do not. However, these studies have been conducted in USA and Europe and may not be applicable to tropical zones.

A Japanese study showed that, in winter, full baths or hot foot baths before bed help people get to sleep quicker and reduce body movements.[22] Some research indicates that about one hour *after* a hot or warm bath, your core body temperature drops slightly, and this temperature decrease is a sleepiness trigger.

Two New York scientists suggest that a rapid decline in core body temperature increases the likelihood of sleepiness signals, and may facilitate the deeper stages of sleep.[23] This sleep laboratory study indicates that core body temperature decreases slightly about 45 minutes before bed, confirming the potential beneficial effects of having a bath *about* one hour before bed — and not having the house heated late in the evening.

I like to go to bed feeling cool and wonder if the world is divided into those who function better when slightly warm and those who prefer to feel cool. You may need to experiment with the temperature of your house and bath to find what works for you.

BEHAVIORAL THERAPY

This therapy involves a therapist helping you change beliefs and attitudes about sleep, establishing better sleep patterns, and eliminating daytime napping. An American study indicates that cognitive behavioral therapy reduces sleep onset and sleep maintenance time by 54 per cent within six weeks.[24]

Sometimes you need to be told many times that you should modify some of your habits for the sake of your health — and you may respond more readily if you pay a lot of money to have a therapist tell you what you already know! The way many of us think and behave is often quite mysterious; however, if your brain has had many repetitions of negative messages, then it may need many repetitions of positive messages to offset these. Have patience with yourself.

BREATHING EXERCISES AND CLEARING NASAL PASSAGES

It is preferable to breathe in through the nostrils because this filters and humidifies the air and helps modify the temperature of the air before it reaches the lungs. If your breathing is impaired you either cannot sleep, or your sleep is not restorative.

A basic breathing technique is as follows:

a) Sit or lie in a comfortable position, with your hands resting lightly on your upper abdomen.

b) As you breathe in through the nose, let your abdomen rise gently.

c) Breathe out through the nose and let the abdomen relax.

d) Simply allow the air to flow gently in and out through your nose, visualize that your upper abdomen is like a soft balloon gently filling with air as you breath in and relaxing as you breath out. To help focus your mind on the breathing, slowly and silently repeat 'in, 2, 3, out, 2, 3' or whatever number is your unforced breathing pace; or you could silently repeat the words 'breathing in, breathing out'. Focusing on the breath can make your chest feel tight if you are anxious, so practice for a few minutes initially and then gradually increase the duration — or use a different strategy. One alternative is to imagine that you are in a peaceful setting such as a church or a rainforest and that you are becoming part of the peaceful atmosphere.

Nasal irrigation before bed can help clear the upper airways and prevent snoring. Yoga suppliers sell 'neti pots' for this purpose or you can use a dropper. You can buy saline solution from a pharmacy or make your own. To make your own saline solution, use 1/3 teaspoon sea salt to 100 ml boiled water, cooled to tepid heat. Saline sprays are easy to use and available from pharmacies.

Caution: If you use a dropper, do not insert it up the nose more than one centimeter. Turn your head to one side and sniff the solution up the nose. With a little practice you will be able to insert two to three droppers full of solution into one nostril, close it with a finger and the solution will run out the other nostril. A little solution will also escape down your throat. When you use solutions in this way the temperature should be tepid so that it feels neither hot nor cold in the nostrils. Do not share these types of remedies otherwise infections may spread.

Other

Health food stores and pharmacies sell inhalers that contain oils such as peppermint, camphor and eucalyptus and I find these convenient to use before bed and when travelling on aeroplanes.

Another option is to hire or buy a negative ionizer. Some of my patients have found these helpful and report that it relaxes the breathing and *seems* to promote restorative sleep.

Depending on the cause and severity of your breathing problem, your practitioner may suggest other options.

HOMEOPATHY

This is a system of natural medicine using tiny doses of remedies that work at a molecular rather than a chemical level. Homeopathic remedies are traditionally matched to the patient's emotional, mental and physical make up. A major advantage of seeing a homeopathic practitioner is that you get a chance to *talk about yourself in detail* — and the practitioner has to listen in order to match you with the most appropriate remedy. There are some homeopathic products that you can buy over-the-counter for insomnia and these often include Coffea, Gelsemium, Urtica and Lobelia, as well as various plant remedies in homeopathic form. Homeopathic remedies can help mild insomnia and are very safe and free of side effects.

HYPNOTHERAPY

My experience is that hypnotherapy can be very helpful for insomnia, as well as alleviating problems linked to poor sleep, such as anxiety and pain. You may wish to discuss the type of hypnotherapy used before paying for a consultation; for example, are you going to be fully awake and aware of what is going on throughout the therapy? My experience is that the type of hypnotherapy used for insomnia is something like a relaxation technique. Some people find that they need to relate to the personality of the therapist or that the sound of the therapist's voice is more important. Therapists' charges are variable so, firstly, check the cost because you may require up to eight sessions.

Simple forms of self-hypnosis include repeating positive statements (affirmations), such as '*I will sleep through the night and wake up refreshed.*' However, for insomniacs indirect suggestions may be more effective, such as '*My eyes are heavy, I'm drifting on a cushion of air*' or '*My body is light, I'm breathing in the soft dark air.*'

MEDITATION

There are many benefits of meditation, including:

•Alleviating insomnia

•Speeding up healing, and helping cope with illnesses

•Increasing learning ability, memory, and immune function

•Harmonizing relationships

•Lowering blood pressure, reducing headaches, reducing asthmatic attacks and reducing seizures

•Reducing anxiety, anger and depression. When you meditate, it's like having a holiday from your problems

•Detoxifying the mind and spirit

People who are calm and positive usually show more activity in the left frontal part of the brain compared to stressed, anxious or depressed people whose right frontal area is more active. It is reasonable to assume that calm, positive people are relatively good sleepers. On the other hand, right frontal types produce more of the stress hormone cortisol and also have fewer natural killer cells that are part of immune resistance to infection and disease. Fearful people tend to have more activity in the part of the brain known as the amygdala. Fears are obviously linked to insomnia.

Twenty-five stressed people undertook an eight-week training course involving 2½ hours of meditation training per week for eight weeks, followed by an all-day silent meditation retreat. Various blood tests were taken before the training as well as EEG tests (brain wave readings). The results were compared to 16 stressed people who did not do the meditation training. The meditators' brains showed a pronounced shift toward the left frontal lobe while non-meditators' brains did not.[25]

Other studies confirm that experienced meditators can deliberately enhance their immune function and switch on the positive part of the brain.

In Eastern traditions, meditation is more or less defined as concentration with a spiritual aim. Physical yoga exercises were *originally* designed to make the body light, flexible and strong so that people seeking spiritual truth could sit comfortably and still in reflection, and ultimately experience the Truth for themselves. A body that is light and strong is able to withstand long periods of meditative searching. The principles behind the physical aspects of yoga include promoting the flow of subtle energies (chakras) to help establish inner peace. Many people find that physical yoga by itself helps relax the body and the mind.

My 25 years' experience as a yoga teacher and practitioner is that *forced* meditation can actually make some people more anxious. Think of your meditation as a holiday and part of your philosophy to enjoy your life.

In some cases before getting into meditation it is better to start with physical and mental relaxation techniques and short periods of concentration. In any event, anxious or agitated people will cope with only 5 — 10 minutes initially and gradually be able to build up to 20 minutes or more.

It has been demonstrated by brain wave tests that if meditators sit quietly and repeat words such as 'dog' or 'cat' this does not have the same effect on the brain as traditional meditation. An Indian study showed that meditators have significantly more alpha brain waves (indicating calmness) and more logical mental functioning than non-meditators.[26]

Meditation techniques include:

•Repeating and thinking about verses from a religious or spiritual text
•Focusing on a light or a symbol, such as the lotus flower, a light, or a spiritual being
•Chanting mantras. This may be done silently and privately, or chanted with a group
•Guided meditation

A sample verse is given below:

The body and the mind are called the field
He who knows this is called the knower of the field.
The wisdom that sees both the field and the knower of the field
is true wisdom and it dwells within every heart,
This true wisdom can enjoy everything
Bhagavad Gita, 13.1-2

After repeating the verse a number of times, you might ask yourself questions such as: What power first drives life on its journey, how am I aware of things, why do I know what is right and what is wrong, and why do I search for truth?

Symbol

The lotus is a common symbol in Eastern beliefs. Followers of Eastern religions and philosophy often touch the 'lotus feet' of the teacher as a mark of respect for the teacher's purity. In bhakti (devotional) yoga, one's chosen ideal or personification of God, is visualized as seated on a lotus or the eyes are compared to the petals of a lotus for their shape and beauty.

The lotus grows in mud but the mud does not taint its flowers and leaves, nor does the water (desires) settle inside the plant. Just as the lotus flower grows in length above the water, a spiritual seeker, though living in the 'muddy waters of the world', aims to keep the mind and heart pure by rising above discord. The lotus flower blooms for a few days only, perhaps symbolizing the transitory nature of human existence; although the plant produces more flowers next season. In yogic philosophy, there is a tiny part of living things that does not die.

In Tantra yoga, the spinal column is associated with non-physical centres of consciousness, each centre (chakra) being represented by a different colored lotus with a certain number of petals. The ultimate chakra is Sahasrarara (just above the top of the head), symbolized by a lotus with a thousand petals, glowing like the moon, bright but gentle, serene and soothing.

You could visualize a lotus flower in the centre of your heart and within that lotus is a tiny space. That tiny space is your everlasting Self — beyond sorrow, old age and death.

If you concentrate on a flower, you are thinking of a flower. If you concentrate on a flower as a symbol of the source of creation then you are meditating.

Mantras

A mantra is a sound, word, phrase or verse that has spiritual significance. Unforced repetition of verses or mantras has been an important meditation technique in India for thousands of years. The word 'Om' is the most common mantra and it represents the Creator and the whole of creation. You could silently repeat the word 'Om' as you breathe in and 'Om' as you breathe out. Eastern mantras are often in the ancient Sanskrit language. Well known mantras are 'Om namah shivaya', 'Om mane padme hum' and the Gayatri mantra. There are hundreds of mantras and these are passed on by teachers, or found in various books, and in various languages. You can buy CDs to learn them.

Guided Meditation

You listen to the words as you are taken on an imaginary spiritual journey. Most guided meditations can be used for relaxation, concentration or meditation and they are somewhat like the technique given in Appendix III.

There are numerous meditation techniques and you may have to try various courses before finding one that suits you. I don't recommend starting with a full weekend of meditation because this may cause discomfort, nor should you commit yourself to large sums of money. However, in Eastern traditions, you are expected to make an offering if there is not a fixed charge.

It may be aggravating for insomniacs to do an activity such as watching the breath repeating to yourself "breathing in, breathing out"; because this may make you over-conscious of your breath and, also, a breathing activity may not be enough to crowd out your anxieties.

Peace of mind comes from developing an appropriate philosophy and compassion for others rather than focusing on yourself but you need to get yourself well before you can help others.

RELAXATION THERAPY

Before relaxing the mind, you may need to begin by relaxing the body and the best way to do this is walking and stretching. Hatha yoga is generally recommended but you need to find a class that suits you. The vigorous physical forms of yoga are too stimulating for insomniacs — especially if the activity is done in the evening.

There are many types of relaxation therapy and you may need to try some different types before you find one that suits you. If you're in a very agitated state, don't try to relax; instead go for a walk, swim or jog.

In Appendix II I have given a standard relaxation therapy that may help reduce anxiety and bedtime agitation. Some people find it helpful if used in conjunction with aromatherapy. The idea is that you use a few drops of the aromatic oils when you listen to the relaxation disk. After a few weeks your brain begins to associate the smell with relaxation, and then you need to use only a few drops of the oil to relax.

Don't be concerned if you can't follow a relaxation program quickly or completely.

SNACKS, BEDTIME

There is no precise evidence relating to foods that promote sleep. It is generally agreed that a large meal before bed worsens insomnia and is not good for your digestion and metabolism. My experience is that you need about three hours' digestive time after a large meal.

If you habitually eat a large meal late in the evening, you may need to change your eating patterns, perhaps by having more food at lunchtime and a late afternoon snack — depending on your work and exercise schedule. Having a healthy late afternoon snack helps maintain your blood sugar level and *may* prevent evening overeating. If you're too busy for lunch and afternoon tea and you work late into the evening, you should evaluate your motives and lifestyle. For whom or what are you a slave? Are you enjoying your life? Given that irregular eating leads to digestive disorders and thickens the blood, are you jeopardizing your health?

Some insomniacs may benefit from a small bedtime snack. This snack must be easily digested and in small quantities but I recommend evening snacks only for those who have an early dinner or those with hypoglycemia (low blood sugar). The brain requires fuel during the night and the body's energy system is driven primarily by glucose and oxygen. Sugary foods are probably the worst snack because they are likely to cause highs and lows rather than an even distribution of glucose. A small quantity of complex carbohydrates, such as whole grains, will produce a more even release of glucose.

Bedtime snacks that may help *some* people include:

- Foods that are rich in essential fatty acids and the best choice would be one to two tablespoons of pepitos (pumpkin seeds). Pumpkin seeds are rich in tryptophan, helpful for prostate enlargement and may help menopause symptoms. Animal studies show that immune suppression due to sleep deprivation can be markedly offset by a diet rich in essential fatty acids.[27] Other foods rich in essential fatty acids that should be included in your meals on a regular basis are oily fish, walnuts, Brazil nuts, flaxseed (linseeds), virgin olive oil, other raw nuts and seeds.

- A few wholegrain biscuits spread with avocado, feta cheese or hummus (chickpea spread)

- About eight olives

- About 3 to 4 tablespoons of plain yoghurt, perhaps with a dessert spoon of pure whey protein mixed through it. (Whey protein is difficult to digest so start with a teaspoon and gradually increase the quantity)

- Lettuce contains the compound lactucin that is sleep inducing. My suggestion is to have a few pieces of cheese wrapped in lettuce leaves. The cheese not only provides tryptophan but is also salty and may help you retain fluid at night; this can reduce nighttime urination. Although a very high salt intake is not recommended, some people go to extremes and if you avoid *all* salty foods this may lead to cramps. I do not add salt to foods and I don't eat many processed foods. However, every day I would have a little of one of the following: miso, Tamari, seaweed or cheese

Some foods and herbs contain melatonin — the sleep hormone. This is a new finding and the purpose of melatonin in plants is to protect against oxidative damage from UV light, drought, extreme temperatures and pollutants. Some researchers say that the melatonin levels in plants are higher at night, others say at flowering, and others say at maturity — but melatonin is also present in seeds, so we will have to wait for more evidence. Studies in animals indicate that melatonin in foods enters the bloodstream and is picked up at binding sites in the brain.[28]

No human studies are available and I doubt that human doses of herbs would supply melatonin in therapeutic quantities. However, ginger is known to contain relatively high levels of melatonin, and this herb is good for your digestion and circulation, so you can only benefit from using it — unless you're allergic to ginger. Have a cup of ginger tea after dinner. Finely chop about a dessert spoon of ginger root; simmer in 1½ cups of water for about eight minutes. Strain and drink. You can adjust the quantity of ginger root to your tolerance and taste. You may sweeten if desired with ½ teaspoon of honey or the naturally sweet herb stevia.

Other common herbs that contain melatonin include St John's wort and feverfew. In one study of Chinese herbs, 64 out of 100 contained melatonin, so it seems likely that numerous foods and herbs contain this hormone.

A US study found that tart cherries (Montmorency and Balaton) contain relatively high levels of melatonin.[29] Cherries are an excellent source of various antioxidants, they contain cancer preventive compounds, they can reduce uric acid levels, they taste nice and they're not fattening. Why not try ½ to 1 cup of cherries after dinner? When cherries are not in season your local health food store should be able to supply you with concentrated cherry juice that does not contain added sugar. I suggest about two tablespoons of cherry juice concentrate daily. Other foods known to contain melatonin are rice, oats and most grains, and probably all fruit and vegetables.

Having a large fluid intake before bed is not recommended because a full bladder will wake you. On the other hand, your mouth and throat tissues may become dry if you become dehydrated and this may wake you. If you are taking remedies just before bed I suggest taking them with about ½ cup of fluid.

Keep bedtime remedies minimal because they can upset the stomach and may be stimulatory for sensitive insomniacs. Aim to get your essential nutrients and beneficial plant compounds by having regular meals and using a wide variety of foods in as natural a state as possible.

Epilogue

There are many sub-groups of insomnia and various causes, and this may explain why some treatments don't work for particular individuals.

You might think that it is too troublesome to change your habits and that a precise regime of sleeping and waking will be a lifelong burden. However, many people find that once they develop a reasonable sleep pattern this has a snowballing effect and healthful sleep allows the brain to regulate total body functioning so that it can cope with the typical ups and downs of everyday life.

Spending hours in bed in the evening *trying* to sleep, or remaining in bed for hours after waking, may disrupt your circadian clock and give your brain the message that bed is for worrying or lolling around rather than for sleeping.

Conflicts within your own mind create disharmony. Don't continue saying that you're going to do or not do something without taking any action, because you are better off enjoying your life instead of berating yourself or feeling negligent.

'Saying' but not 'doing' creates disharmony within yourself. You might desire to stay up late at night drinking and looking at TV but feel that this compromises your health; or your work and family commitments require that you get up early, and then you feel irritable or guilty during the day. Yet, when night comes you feel good and resist bed. Your mind has linked feeling good to late nights. A solution may be to find a job that allows you to start later in the morning but most employers are not that flexible and this regime may be at odds with your family's program. Perhaps find a middle course by having less stimulation after dinner, getting up somewhat earlier and gradually getting to bed somewhat earlier. Another theory is that if you go to bed even later, this will make you so tired that you'll eventually get to bed earlier — but meantime you will be very sleep-deprived.

Not many people have the option of joining the night people. There are plenty of them on talk back radio, in clubs and hotels — and shift workers.

Famous Insomniacs

The list includes Thomas Edison, Napoleon, Margaret Thatcher, Van Gogh, Benjamin Franklin, Charles Dickens, Oscar Wilde, Lewis Carroll, and many well-known authors, philosophers, politicians, entertainers and inventors. You will note that some of these people did not come to a good end!

You may have read that Albert Einstein never slept more than an hour or two at a time, others report that he slept for nine hours or more. In any event, he performed exceedingly well at mathematics and physics, received many awards, played the violin, was politically active, and lived for 76 years — and had somewhere between two to nine hours sleep every 24 hours!

The total number of hours people sleep every 24 hours is not a measurement of their nobility.

Appendix I

RESOURCES AND FURTHER READING

I give below a small selection of the many centres and products available for poor sleepers and their bed partners:

•A useful Australian site: http://www.med.monash.edu.au/medicine/alfred
Explains different types of snoring and lists information about The Alfred Sleep Disorders & Ventilatory Failure Service.

•Sleep and common sleep disorders. The Victorian Government Better Health Channel
http://www.betterhealth.vic.gov.au/bhcv2/bhcarticles.nsf/pages/Sleep_ and_common_sleep_disorders

•Child and Youth Health: Information for parents, Child and Youth Health, Government of South Australia
http://www.cyh.com/cyh/youthtopics/usr_srch2.stm?topic_ id=1619&precis=null.

•Obstructive sleep apnoea, The Australian Lung Foundation
http://www.nevdgp.org.au/geninf/lung_f/sleep-apnoea.health.html

If you do a general Internet search of 'apnoea', 'snoring' or 'insomnia' you will find a long list of sources, including sleep clinics in Australia and overseas. Here are a few examples:

•The insomnia bookstore: http://www.neuronic.com/insomnia_bookstore. htm
Lists many books and alternative remedies

•The Sleep Medicine Home Page: http://www.users.cloud9.net/~thorpy
Provides sleep-related news, lists discussion groups, and covers sleep disorders, professional associations and organisations, journals and books, sleep research sites, and education sites.

- The National Sleep Foundation, USA. http://www.sleepfoundation.org
  A nonprofit, independent organization dedicated to research and providing information to the general public.

- Sleep and other health problems: http://www.drgreene.com/21_617.html
  Practical answers for a long list of specific problems.

- http:///store.yahoo.com/earplugstore/index.htlm?ESCOM+Forward
  Different types of earplugs including an in-ear white noise machine purported to give protection against the loudest snorer!

- Snoring problems: http://www.quietnitecap.com/nav.html
  Helpful hints, healthy breathing, famous snorers, jokes and a support for the jaw to control snoring.

- Light therapy: http://www.sltbr.org
  Society for Light Treatment and Biological Rhythms

- www.ZenSleepinfo
  This is a completely different way of looking at sleep not from the point of view of trying to obtain it but to escape from how you perceive sleep and learning from your own direct observation. Does your own mind create suffering, do you have to sleep well to perform well and be successful?

- Federation of international sleep organizations: http://www.wfsrs.org
  Information mainly for practitioners.

- The American Academy of Sleep Medicine: http://www.aasmnet.org
  Provides lists of other websites.

If you want to do your own scientific research of sleep disorders, there are a number of scientific journals devoted solely to sleep research, although if you are a poor sleeper this may give your brain too many insomnia messages. Some of the journals are listed below:

Journal of Sleep Research
Sleep
Sleep & Breathing
Sleep Medicine
Sleep Medicine Reviews

There are other medical and scientific journals that contain sleep research including *Journal of Pineal Research* and *Journal of Biological Rhythms*.

Books, Audio Books, CDs, Cassettes

Your local library or bookshop may be able to help you and there are some specialist suppliers:

- Pauline Books & Media supply Christian books, CDs and cassettes and they have stores in Sydney, Melbourne and Adelaide. They also have a detailed website and a mail order service. http://www.paulinebooks.com.au

- Adyar Bookshop has over 45,000 books, CDs and cassettes on just about every belief system and alternative therapy. If you live in Sydney you can visit the store at 230 Clarence Street. It doesn't have a full printed catalogue but you can get on the mailing list for book news or visit the website at www.adyar.com.au

- Southern Scene Pty Ltd is a specialist supplier of large print and audio books. It is located at 47-49 Kingsway, Kingsgrove NSW 2208, and the website is www.southernscene.com.au

- ABC Shops and Centres abcshop.com.au, or phone 1300 360 111. The ABC has a wide selection of audio material that may be useful for insomnia in general and also as 'sound diversion' for tinnitus sufferers.

Sleep Disorders Centres In Australia

- White Pages — see 'Sleep Apnea/Apnoea'. Under this heading you will also find equipment suppliers.

- Yellow Pages — under Medical Practitioners see 'Sleep Disorders' and 'Sleep Apnoea'.

- Most large hospitals have specialised sleep clinics, but you need a medical practitioner referral for a consultation.

There are also Sleep Laboratories and Sleep Monitoring Units where people can get diagnosed. In these specialised centres you can be monitored in various ways including measurements of brain waves, air flow, blood oxygen, hormone levels, eye movements, muscle tension, movements and heart activity. You will need a doctor's referral to be tested in a sleep laboratory. I highly recommend these diagnostic sleep laboratories for people who are unable to sleep for unknown reasons, particularly where they awaken exhausted or find themselves falling asleep inappropriately during the day.

A STANDARD RELAXATION THERAPY

You can record this for your self.

There's no particular magic in the words and you can change them. Make your disk when you feel relaxed and don't worry about the sound of your voice. It is important to speak slowly and rhythmically because when you listen to your recording, this sends relaxing messages to the brain and body. At the end of your recording you could fill the remainder of your disk with some music or sounds from a relaxation CD.

If you fall asleep before the recording is finished your machine will switch off at the end. Some people say that you absorb the relaxation effects even though you are asleep and not conscious of the words.

This particular program may be done in conjunction with sedative aromatic oils — for example: lavender by itself or combined with blue chamomile and marjoram oils. Before starting the cassette put about 1 to 2 drops of the oil under your nose. When you are listening to the words, your ears send the oral message to your brain at the same time as your nose sends the odor message. Studies show that after a week or so your brain associates the particular smell with relaxation — and then you need only a few drops of the oils to get a restful night's sleep.

Get everything ready for bed before starting the disk.

The recording:

I will focus on the words, silently repeating each phrase.

If any thoughts interrupt my concentration, I'll simply observe them. Then I will return to concentrating on the words.

My breath is flowing gently in and out through the nostrils
I will silently repeat each phrase
Any sounds from outside or inside are gently washing over me
My body and mind will rest as much as they need to
If there's an emergency I will wake up

My breath is flowing gently and naturally
In and out through the nostrils
As I breathe in I say to myself the word 'om'
As I breathe out I count silently and slowly

Om 1, Om 2, Om 3, Om 4, Om 5, Om 6, Om 7, Om 8, Om 9, Om 10, Om 11, Om 12, Om 13, Om 14, Om 15, Om 16, Om 17, Om 18, Om 19, Om 20.

My feet are soft and relaxed
My legs are soft and relaxed
Buttocks and lower abdomen soft and relaxed

Breathing in the dark soft air
Lower back is soft and relaxed
Upper back soft and relaxed
Chest is soft and relaxed

I breathe in calmness, I exhale peace
I breathe in calmness, I exhale peace

The fingers of my right hand are soft and relaxed
My right hand is soft and relaxed
Right arm and right shoulder relax

The fingers of my left hand are soft and relaxed
My left hand is soft and relaxed
Left arm and left shoulder relax

Breathing in the dark soft air

My throat is soft and relaxed
I breathe in calmness, I exhale peace
I breathe in calmness, I exhale peace

Back of the neck relax
Back of the head relax
Top of the head relax
My forehead is smooth and calm
Eyes are gently closed like soft black velvet

I breathe in calmness, I exhale peace
I breathe in calmness, I exhale peace

I know that worry is a futile emotion
And even if I worry ten times more, I won't change the situation
I can't control my thoughts because
I don't know where they come from
If any unwanted thoughts come to my mind
I'll calmly observe them
Then I will focus on the words

As I breathe out I let go
I'm merging into the soft dark air

Hidden deep within me there is a wise inner self
When I sleep MY wise inner self looks after me
I know that worry is a futile emotion

My wise inner self is calm and peaceful
Nothing can harm my wise inner self
Everything is soft, comfortable and safe
I'm merging into the soft dark air

My body and mind will rest as long as they need to
My body is like soft, dark velvet
I'm merging into the soft, dark, air

Breathe in calmness, exhale peace
Breathe in calmness, exhale peace

Everything is relaxed and safe
My body merges into the soft, dark velvety air

I'm drifting into the soft, dark, velvety air

My body is soft and relaxed
My mind is clear and calm
I'm merging into the soft darkness
I'm drifting into the gentle darkness
Everything is soft and peaceful

Om 1, Om 2, Om 3, Om 4, Om 5, Om 6, Om 7, Om 8, Om 9, Om 10, Om 11, Om 12, Om 13, Om 14, Om 15, Om 16, Om 17, Om 18, Om 19, Om 20.

NOTE

The word Om has no meaning but it is a universal, spiritual sound symbol, signifying ONENESS. It represents the universe — from the Creator to the tiniest particle and includes all living beings, things and thoughts.

Appendix III

A GUIDED RELAXATION TECHNIQUE FOR REDIRECTING YOUR THOUGHTS

If you have multiple thoughts racing through your head or a strong emotional feeling, a simple technique such as repeating the word 'om' or relaxation music may not occupy enough mental space in your brain to offset unwanted thoughts.

The aim is to *record* the words *when you are feeling relaxed*, saying each phrase slowly and calmly — with a gap in between each phrase — so that when you listen to the words, you can silently repeat them as you visualize the scene. You then use this disk just before bed or in bed. I find it helpful if I tell myself that I'm going to listen to every word to the end of the tape — and then I rarely hear the end!

The recording:

I picture myself in a beautiful, soft green rain forest
Everything is calm and peaceful
The foliage of the tall trees blocks out the sunlight
The temperature is perfect
Everything is calm, soft and dark
Nearby is a gentle stream
The water is clear and pure, and gently trickling over the rocks
I'm lying comfortably picturing the peaceful, healing surroundings
Breathing in the pure, soft air
Picturing the moss, ferns and shrubs that surround the stream
And the tall, soft green rainforest trees

My body is light and comfortable
I breathe in the pure, peaceful atmosphere
Picturing the clear water of the gentle stream
And the soft green of the moss, ferns, shrubs and trees
Green is the centre of the color spectrum
It is the color of harmony and balance
Picturing the soft green of the moss, ferns, shrubs and trees
Why is this rainforest so pure and peaceful?
Why is it so rich and green?

When the rain comes, the earth receives the refreshing water
The earth doesn't examine the water, it accepts it
When the leaves fall, the plants use the fallen leaves to nourish themselves
The plants don't criticise the leaves, they simply take them in as nourishment

In the same way, I will not worry about everyday happenings
If everything went smoothly day after day I'd complain of boredom
I think of myself as a giant fig tree
I started my life as a tiny seed
I grew out of the darkness of the soil and up towards the light
My roots are firm and strong
My branches are diverse and spreading

I take in the light through my leaves
My bark protects me
My roots take in water and nourishment
I experience the universe
I sway in the wind but am not broken
Through my leaves I provide life-giving oxygen
I cool the air, intercept the rain, and buffer the wind
I provide shade for smaller plants
I give food and shelter without question to all living creatures
I prevent erosion, and I store water
I purify the air

All this I do without charge 24 hours a day, year after year
Without moving, without payment and with barely a sound
Insects chew my leaves, birds peck at my bark
People trample over my roots
The wind takes some of my leaves, but I grow new leaves
I remain patient, persistent, enduring and adaptable
I am part of the universe

I do not criticise or blame
My true nature is generous, forgiving, calm and peaceful
I observe everything but remain calm and peaceful
Calm and peaceful

I am not suggesting that you should completely avoid thinking about your problems because this is how you may eventually resolve them, however, if you are an insomniac you should be aware that excessive dwelling on your worries only increases them — and nighttime worrying needs to be restricted. Generally, my recommendation is to set a time during the day to focus on your problems and this focusing becomes harmful only if the problems take an excessive amount of time, or if you keep going over the same thing without coming to any solution or acceptance, or if your worries interfere with your daily life and sleep.

You need to *think* because conscious thought is your propelling force and you also need a belief that you have the power to make positive changes. If you tell yourself you cannot do anything to improve your situation, then you are adding another negative message into your brain. Of course, we all have some failures and backsliding but these can be offset by awareness that you are taking steps to get more happiness and peace.

MEDICATIONS FOR SLEEPING AND DEPRESSION

This book's primary aim is to discuss holistic solutions for those with sleep disorders and insomnia. It would not be complete without a discussion of the pros and cons of pharmaceutical treatments for insomnia.

One must sleep and if sleep becomes impossible for whatever reason it is good to know that modern pharmaceutical drugs have come a long way. Prolonged and/or total inability to sleep can lead to a stress breakdown and vice versa. Sleep is like a safety valve on the high pressure machine of your mind – when the pressure is about to rupture the machine we need to look into using drugs to salvage our nervous system and sanity. Thank God these medications are there because they can be life saving and of course allow you to continue to function and perform, often at a fairly high level.

In general it is best to have the philosophy that you will only need the drugs until the stress and difficulties subside or even better go away and thankfully they often do, as human beings are remarkably adaptable. Some of us inherit a very sensitive or worrying disposition and this makes us more vulnerable to stress induced insomnia. The nervous system can be compared to the strings on a violin and when the strings are pulled too tight they can snap and break; this is where the drugs come in, as they re-tune the strings and allow the music to play again in harmony.

With my patients I always tell them that the medication I prescribe is to help them get over the worst of the stressful situation and when they are feeling back in control and able to sleep again, we will try to slowly reduce the dosage of the drugs. This may take only a few months or sometimes up to several years. However if we aim to use the smallest dose that works it is much easier to gradually withdraw the drugs completely. It is often surprising to find that very small doses of medications can be effective for insomnia, which shows us that the power of positive thought is very important. This was seen in the case of my own sister Madeleine who averted a stress breakdown in herself by using a ¼ of a sleeping tablet every night until her enormous work load of being a carer for several people eased off.

I always try to prescribe antidepressant drugs in preference to sleeping pills (sedative drugs), as the antidepressant drugs are not really addictive or habit forming. Conversely sleeping tablets or sedatives are habit forming.

Many people hold the misconception that antidepressant drugs are highly addictive and to take them is an admission of a weakness of character; however they primarily act on a chemical imbalance, that under severe stress may be impossible to overcome by will power and natural supplements alone. After all what we all seek is a better quality of life as we are not on the planet for very long!

PRESCRIBED MEDICATIONS AND SLEEP

So when should you see a doctor or pharmacist to discuss medication for sleep? You may need medication if...

- Insomnia is interfering with your quality of life and natural therapies combined with improvements in diet and life style have failed

- Insomnia is part of a known medical condition

- Your insomnia is a condition by itself and is chronic and could lead to a nervous breakdown, severe depression, anxiety attacks or inability to function

Table of different Anti Depressant Drugs

CLASS	DRUG	SEDATING Effect	Comments
TRICYCLIC antidepressants	Amitryptyline - Tryptanol Doxepin - Sinequan Imipramine Clomipramine Desipramine	++++ ++++ +++ +++ +	• Relieves panic attack & depression • Low doses are effective for chronic pain, fibromyalgia & irritable bladder • Weight gain, dry mouth & constipation are side effects of high doses
SSRI - Selective Serotonin Reuptake Inhibitors	Fluvoxamine - Luvox Citalopram- Cipramil Sertraline - Zoloft Paroxetine –Aropax Fluoxetine – Prozac Escitalopram – Lexapro	+ – + + – –	• Generally safe & well tolerated • Discontinuation syndrome may be a problem • When first prescribed may cause agitation & insomnia
SNRI - Serotonin & Noradrenalin Reuptake Inhibitors	Venlafaxine –Efexor	+	• Dry mouth & sometimes sedating Effective in severe depression

CLASS	DRUG	SEDATING Effect	Comments
RIMA - Reversible inhibitor of MAO	Moclobemide – Aurorix	–	• May cause insomnia and headaches • Helpful in depression where fatigue & weight gain are a problem
NaSSA - Noradrenalin Serotonin specific Antidepressants	Mirtazapine Avanza/Remeron	++	• Weight gain is common • Effective for depression & insomnia
NARI - Noradrenalin Reuptake Inhibitors	Reboxetine - Edronax	–	• Effective for severe depression but may aggravate insomnia
MAOI - Monoamine Oxidase Inhibitors	Phenelzine - Nardil Tranylcypromine –Parnate	–	• Serious drug and food interactions • May cause agitation and insomnia • Effective for severe depression

Insomnia is often related to important psychological conditions such as depression and anxiety, and these should be treated as a priority, as the sleep tends to improve as the underlying disorder improves. Sometimes insomnia occurs by itself and careful use of medication must be discussed with your doctor.

DEPRESSION AND ANXIETY

Sleep disorder is a primary symptom of depression and lack of sleep can cause depression!

The very common condition known as major depressive disorder has as one of its primary features a persistent disturbance of sleep. Depressed people begin to wake regularly at 2 or 3 a.m. and find it very difficult to drift off again. They may be very agitated or very slow and miserable. Their thoughts may scatter or centre obsessively on one topic over and over; they just can't get back to sleep! Others may find that worry and whirling thoughts make it difficult to get off to sleep at their regular bedtime. Other depressed patients sleep too much, nap through the day, and can't get moving! This especially occurs in depressed young adults.

The depressive disorders affect about 25% of women and 20% of men at some time in their lives. They are caused by wiring and chemical imbalances in the brain. Other typical symptoms of a depressive illness include loss of interest and motivation, poor concentration, sad or depressed mood and weight changes, most commonly loss of weight.

The tendency for depression is genetically determined and causes the brain to run like a faulty battery, which gradually discharges and becomes flat.

ANXIETY DISORDERS are also known to interfere with sleep. Panic disorder often causes people to wake in the full throes of a panic attack, with intense fear, rapid breathing and heart beat, and a feeling of imminent doom! This can occur several times during one night and may even be associated with gastrointestinal symptoms such as vomiting or diarrhoea attacks. Post traumatic stress disorder is another type of anxiety and often features terrifying recurrent nightmares. Others with generalized anxiety disorder (GAD) find it hard to get to sleep, as they are worrying about everything!

ANTIDEPRESSANT DRUGS AND SLEEP

Both depression and anxiety disorders are commonly treated with antidepressants, which are drugs that modify the chemicals (neuro-transmitters) in the brain.

The antidepressant drugs gradually change the brain's chemical imbalance leading to an improvement in sleep, usually within a few short weeks. Unfortunately experience with these medications has shown that the antidepressants may also cause insomnia in some people, especially if they are used for too long. And whilst the mood has improved, sometimes healthy balanced sleep remains a problem. If this occurs in your case, the doctor can change your medication, or better still very slowly reduce the dose and often have success with sleep. Sometimes it is necessary to add on other medications ("augmentation") for a short term period in order to get that precious time out in sleep!

Most depressed patients are commenced on the drugs known as Selective Serotonin Re-uptake Inhibitors (SSRIs) in the first instance when depression is the cause of sleeplessness. Mirtazapine (Avanza) may also be used and is often quite sedating early in treatment. In the range of the SSRI medications, fluvoxamine , sertraline and paroxetine are more likely to promote sleep earlier in the treatment. Fluoxetine(Prozac/Lovan) may be more activating and is good for depression with hypersomnia, that is oversleeping.

Quite separately to anxiety and depression, you may be offered an antidepressant drug to treat insomnia due to other causes. Low doses of some antidepressants, especially the Tricyclic class of drugs, will cause night time sedation, but not be strong enough to treat depression or anxiety disorders. These LOW DOSES can be most helpful for some patients with severe chronic insomnia but no other apparent symptoms of anxiety or depression. Interestingly the Tricyclic drugs can also help some insomniacs whose chronic pain is keeping them from sleeping restfully. They are commonly prescribed for chronic pain of various causes, including shingles, neuralgia and fibromyalgia, as well as other conditions such as migraine and tension headache. In such cases they can be very effective at promoting a deep restorative sleep. The Tricyclic drugs can also be used effectively to overcome irritable bladder and nocturnal urinary frequency, and nocturnal diarrhoea due to an overactive bowel. The Tricyclic drugs can prevent panic attacks from disrupting sleep and are far more effective and safer than sedatives or sleeping pills.

Different families of antidepressant drugs exist, and over many years, new classes have been discovered, all of which work on brain chemistry in different ways (see table on page 158). One of the common properties of all antidepressants is to restore the "sleep-wake" cycle. Most people treated at adequate doses, for several weeks are eventually able to enjoy more restful nights! Check the table to see which antidepressants are more likely to have a sedative effect. Individual people respond very differently to these medications, so the table demonstrates general trends only.

Your doctor will guide you as to which drug is likely to help you the most with minimal side effects. This will depend on the cause of your insomnia. There is no magic recipe to determine which drug is best for you. Research may one day guide doctors as to which chemical is most disordered and which medication is most likely to help. Meanwhile, for most people with insomnia due to anxiety or depression, it is a case of trial and error. Many patients may need to try more than one drug to find the one that is right for them. But the good news is that over 80% of patients will respond to medication for depression and anxiety when psychological treatment and/or natural therapies are not enough.

Eventually after 2 - 4 weeks and sometimes less, the sleep cycle improves in most cases, the worries recede and positive feelings and mental drive return.

Because it takes time for anti-depressant drugs to normalize brain chemistry, some acutely disturbed patients may need *short term* treatment with other medications, called HYPNOTICS or ANXIOLYTICS, (and commonly known as sleeping pills or sleeping tablets), to be able to turn off the negative, fearful and worrying thoughts long enough to get off to sleep.

ADVERSE EFFECTS OF ANTIDEPRESSANT DRUGS

Generally speaking the antidepressant drugs are well tolerated however they must be prescribed very carefully, especially in patients who are in a highly stressed or agitated state. Generally speaking they should be *commenced* in a small dose – for example ¼ of a tablet daily for the first few days, and then ½ a tablet daily for another week, and then one tablet daily. This is the best way to avoid side effects.

The best known example of the antidepressant drugs is the original SRI drug called Prozac. Indeed there is a very interesting book written by the American psychiatrist Peter D. Kramer, titled *"Listening to Prozac"*, published by Penguin.

Using Prozac as an example, the following is a summary of its potential problems:

- •May cause anxiety, insomnia, altered appetite and weight loss, may activate mania/hypomania, or seizures.

- •Very close monitoring is required if there is a suicidal tendency.

- •It may reduce blood sodium levels in the elderly, and cause reduced platelet function (easy bruising/bleeding).

- •It can impair kidney and liver function and is not recommended during pregnancy and lactation.

Other adverse effects are possible and include:

Weakness, sensitivity to the sun, allergies, headache, palpitations, low blood pressure, diarrhoea, nausea, vomiting, dyspepsia, anorexia, weight loss or weight gain, easy bruising, twitching, anxiety, dizziness, abnormal dreams, decreased libido, impotence, inability to orgasm, nervousness, sleep disorders, abnormal thinking, yawning, muscle spasm, itching, rashes, sweating, hair loss and changes of personality.

There are other problems not listed in reference books and these should be considered. For example, you can have too much serotonin and symptoms of this include sweating, confusion, high temperature, rigid arms and legs, and occasionally, seizures, coma and death. This is called "serotonin syndrome" and may be brought about by very high doses of antidepressants, interactions with other medications such as anti-migraine and anti-smoking drugs, and by social drugs. Combining antidepressants with St John's wort and tryptophan may trigger similar symptoms. It is unlikely that excess serotonin could be triggered by foods, herbs, and natural supplements — at least at normal intakes or label doses.

May cause serious, sometimes fatal reactions, if taken with other types of antidepressants such as monoamine oxidase inhibitors. This is rare and should not occur if you are under the regular care of a psychiatrist.

ANXIOLYTICS AND HYPNOTICS (SLEEPING PILLS)

The term "anxiolytic" means anxiety reducing and the term "hypnotic" means sleep inducing.
Most of these drugs do both, and are commonly prescribed as *short term* sleeping aids or as treatments for severe anxiety. Sleeping pills can be useful when chronic anxiety prevents sleep but I prefer the tricyclic antidepressant drugs as they control chronic anxiety, panic attacks and promote sleep and are not addictive. Sleeping pills can be used for short term insomnia on

an occasional basis. These drugs require a doctor's prescription and many doctors are understandably reluctant to prescribe them because of the potential of side effects and dependency.

Benzodiazepines

Short and long-acting benzodiazepines, used to treat anxiety and other psychiatric conditions, are also helpful in treating some sleep disorders. Unfortunately all benzodiazepines are habit-forming and more or less physically addictive. But they do induce sleep! They are only to be used as *short-term treatment*.

Rebound insomnia occurs when a patient stops taking sleeping pills such as benzodiazepine medication, and the patient will experience several nights of insomnia that are much worse than they experienced before treatment was prescribed. These medications should not be used alone to treat depression and/or insomnia.

Examples of benzodiazepine drugs include Temaze, Normison, Halcion, Serepax, Valium, Mogadon and Xanax. Their generic names include alprazolam, oxazepam, diazepam, temazepam, triazolam clonazepam and nitrazepam.

Non-benzodiazepine sleeping pills include zopiclone (Imovane) and zolpidem (Stilnox), which may still be addictive in longer term use.

Actions of hypnotics (sleeping pills)

•Shorten the time it takes to fall asleep

•Increase total sleep time

•Decrease how often you wake

•Give you a rest while awaiting the effect of other treatments, eg antidepressant therapy if depression underlies insomnia

How long should drug treatment last?

- Accepted insomnia guidelines call for short-term treatment, but long-term use of sleeping pills is not uncommon.

- Four weeks is the recommended limit.

- *Refusing* to prescribe hypnotics may cause unnecessary patient distress, particularly when the person does well on the same dose and has *no* side effects.

- Most sleep specialists share the belief that sleeping pills should not be a long-term answer to poor sleep for most people who have trouble sleeping.

Substances that can interfere with prescribed sleeping tablets include:

Over-the-counter sleep medicines such as anti-histamines, valerian, cannabis, pain killers, other prescribed dugs and alcohol can all interact adversely with prescribed sleeping tablets and greatly increase their side effects.

Side effects of sleeping pills (hypnotics) include-

- Daytime sleepiness

- Forgetfulness and mental confusion

- Higher risk of falling and causing injury, especially in older people

- Inability to drive safely

Withdrawal symptoms:

These can occur when the sleeping pills are stopped and include –

Anxiety, panic attacks, insomnia, nightmares, headaches, low mood and shivering, sweating, convulsive disorders in patients with epilepsy. Sleeping tablets may cause problems in addictive-prone people because benzodiazepines can lead to addiction. Total time for withdrawal varies from 4 — 16 weeks

166

Sleeping pills are basically central nervous system depressants; they can distort the way you perceive sleep and they wipe out part of your sleep process, such as REM cycles. That is why you can experience vivid dreams and nightmares when you stop taking them.

In the light of the known adverse effects, it is not surprising that a British victim of over-prescription of Valium has set up a website with over 450 pages of information about tranquillizers [1] One study of long-term benzodiazepine users found that supervised tapering down, along with cognitive behavioral therapy was very helpful in lowering sleeping pill use although sleep improvements may become noticeable only after several months of benzodiazepine abstinence.[2]

OVER-THE-COUNTER MEDICATIONS

Some sleep medications are sold over the counter (OTC) without a prescription in pharmacies and supermarkets and can be quite effective for many insomniacs. If you take OTC products for sleep, use them carefully and watch for side effects because they may make you drowsy the next day.

Antihistamine drugs block chemicals released during allergy attacks and are commonly prescribed for allergies, itchy rashes, hives and hay fever. Many antihistamines have a sedating effect. These products may not be safe to take if you are/or plan to become pregnant or are breastfeeding, you regularly drink alcohol, or take other medications that have sedating effects including antidepressants. Older people should also be careful, as should those with untreated sleep apnoea. People with glaucoma, chronic bronchitis, obstructive airways disease, and prostate gland problems should not take antihistamine drugs. Examples of antihistamine drugs include Polaramine, Phenergan, Vallergan, Zadine and Unisom.

Other sedating OTC drugs include doxylamine, available as Restavit or Mersyndol.

Appendix V

SLEEP SCIENCE

Your circadian or biological sleep clock is a pair of pinhead-sized structures that contain about 20,000 brain cells that control your sleep-wake cycle. These 'clock cells' are located in the brain's hypothalamus — specifically the suprachiasmic nucleus, just above the point where the optic nerves cross (see page 11). Light that reaches the retina at the back of the eye causes signals to travel along the optic nerves to the circadian sleep clock. Signals are then relayed to various parts of the brain including the pineal gland, which produces the sleep hormone melatonin. Melatonin begins to increase after darkness falls. The 'clock cells' also control functions that are synchronised with sleeping and waking such as core body temperature, urine production, secretion of various hormones and changes in blood pressure.

There are various external cues (zeitgebers) that adjust your circadian sleep clock, such as the timing of your meals and temperature. However, light is the most important influence and explains why about 77 per cent of blind people with no perception of light have abnormal circadian rhythms and sleep problems, while those with light perception sleep better.[1] When totally blind people are given 5 mg melatonin one hour before bedtime this increases total sleep time and sleep efficiency.[2] It might help the circadian rhythm of some blind people if they go outside in the early morning light without glasses and with their arms and legs exposed to the light because some research suggests there may be 'clock cells' in parts of the body other than the brain. In any event, early morning outdoor activity has the benefit of physical activity as well as providing natural vitamin D at a time when sunlight is not harmful to the skin.

Stages Of Sleep And Their Function

REM (rapid eye movement) sleep resembles wakefulness and this is the period linked to recallable dreams. REM sleep initially lasts about 20 minutes but becomes longer as the night wears on and this 'active' sleep occurs about every 90 minutes in adults — and somewhat less in children.

It is now known that we also dream during slow wave (nonREM) sleep, although we don't normally remember these dreams. We also dream during the day — although we are not usually conscious of this because there are too many other things happening. Dreaming is an interesting part of human functioning but the dreams may or may not have much significance and dream interpretation seems to be largely guesswork unless linked to trauma or major stress.

REM sleep stimulates brain regions used in learning and it is especially important for the brain development of infants — who have much more REM sleep than adults. Studies show that REM sleep affects some types of learning because people deprived of REM sleep cannot recall what they learned.

Animal studies show that exposure to a novel, enriched environment causes the brain to turn on a gene called zif-268 during subsequent REM sleep. This gene turns on after heightened brain activity and is associated with strengthened communication between nerve cells in different parts of the brain, and this provides an explanation of how the sleeping brain consolidates recently formed memories. I think this indicates that your brain likes new experiences and learning, although no doubt there is a point at which too much learning may create too much excitement — and perhaps disordered REM sleep. Zif-268 is turned off during slow wave sleep. However, during slow wave sleep there is reactivation of brain circuits (hippocampal-neocorticol) that were activated during waking and learning —

and, it is known that in REM sleep there is consolidation of this new learning into long-term memory.[3]

Another suggested function of REM sleep is that the watery liquid behind the cornea of the eye needs to circulate to bring oxygen to the cornea. When the eyelids are closed during sleep, the circulation slows dramatically but the rapid eye movements increase activity to prevent corneal suffocation.

Both REM sleep and slow wave sleep are associated with increased production of proteins, your cells' building blocks.

During stage two of nonREM sleep, (also called slow wave, delta wave or quiet sleep) there is distinctive rapid brain wave activity known as sleep spindles. In stage three there are very slow delta brain waves and some spindle activity and stage four is almost all delta wave. It is usually difficult to wake someone in stages three and four, commonly called deep sleep.

Sleep Abnormalities

Extreme early risers (larks) have a condition called 'advanced sleep-phase syndrome' which means that they feel sleepy very early in the evening and consequently they wake very early; and they may be frustrated as they wait for others to wake. Extreme owls have 'delayed sleep-phase syndrome' and they are simply unable to go to sleep if they go to bed at 10 p.m.

Both categories may be able to modify their sleep pattern; however it may take months, even years, to modify sleeping habits and it is unlikely that an extreme lark would become an extreme owl. In some cases these sleep syndromes are genetic but bear in mind that lifestyle habits may be inherited.

There are specific categories of sleep disorders, called parasomnias that involve unwanted physical or behavioral occurrences during sleep. Rapid eye movement (REM) sleep behavior disorders and slow wave sleep disorders may occur in healthy people, during stressful times and in those with neurological conditions, but they are not linked to psychiatric (mental) illnesses. While we sleep our brain maintains our heart and breathing but our skeletal muscles are toned down. Parasomnias may manifest as physically acting out dreams, talking, kicking, punching, sleep walking, and even complex activity such as dressing. Usually the individual has no memory of the activity upon waking.

Although sleep deprivation may be a cause of parasomnias and other problems that occur during sleep, this book is not about parasomnias, night seizures and major disorders, as these require medical diagnosis and practitioner treatment.

Hypersomnia means excess sleep, either at night or during the day. An adult requiring more than ten hours sleep a night should get practitioner advice. Excessive sleepiness can have many causes including diseases such as low thyroid, depression, various pharmaceutical and other drugs, and emotional conflict causing a desire to escape through sleep. Narcolepsy, is a rare disorder where people fall asleep inappropriately, lose muscle control and dream during the day.

A number of studies mentioned in this book have been conducted in sleep laboratories using polysomnography. A polysomnogram is a simultaneous recording of various activities related to sleep and wakefulness.

- Electrodes on the scalp monitor brain waves that indicate levels of wakefulness and sleep.

- Electrodes on the skin around the eyes monitor eye movements.

- Electrodes on the skin on various part of the body measure muscle movement and twitching.

- It is also possible to measure heart, pulse, breathing, core body temperature and so on.

REFERENCES

INTRODUCTION

1. Masaya T. 'The role of prescribed napping in sleep medicine', Sleep Medicine Reviews, 7; 227-35: 2003.

CHAPTER 1

1. Means MK, Edinger JD, Glenn DM, Fins AI. 'Accuracy of sleep perceptions among insomnia sufferers and normal sleepers', *Sleep Medicine*, 4; 285:96: 2003.

2. Van Dongen HP, Maislin G, Mullington JM, Dinges DF. 'The cumulative cost of additional wakefulness: dose-response effects on neurobehavioral functions and sleep physiology from chronic sleep restriction and total sleep deprivation', *Sleep*, 26; 117-27: 2003.

3. Carskadan MA, Harvey K, Duke P, Anders TF, Litt IF, Dement WC. 'Pubertal changes in daytime sleepiness', *Sleep*: 2; 453-60: 1980.

4. Dick DJ, Duffy JF, Czeisler CA. 'Contribution of circadian physiology and sleep homeostasis to age-related changes in human sleep', *Chronobiology International*, 17; 286-311: 2000.

5. Garfinkel D, Laudon M, Nof D, Zisapel N. 'Improvement of sleep quality in elderly people by controlled-release melatonin', *Lancet*, 346; 541-4: 1995.

CHAPTER 2

1. Stickgold R, Whidbee D, Schirmer B, Patel V, Hobson JA. 'Visual discrimination task improvement: a multi-step process occurring during sleep', *Journal of Cognitive Neuroscience*, 12; 246-54: 2000.

2. Gais S, Plihal W. Wagner U, Born J. 'Early sleep triggers memory for early visual discrimination skills', *Nature Neuroscience*, 3; 1335-9: 2000.

3. Roge J, Pebayle T, El Hannachi S, Muzet A. 'Effect of sleep deprivation and driving duration on the useful visual field in younger and older subjects during simulator driving', *Vision Research*, 43; 1465-72: 2003.

4. Rajaratnam SM, Arendt J. 'Health in a 24-h society', *Lancet*, 358; 999-1005: 2001.

5. Rowley J. 'Insomnia', http://www.emedicine.com/MED/topic2698.htm.

6. Kripke DF, Garfinkel L, Wingard DL, Klauber MR, Marler MR. 'Mortality associated with sleep duration and insomnia', *Archives of General Psychiatry*, 59; 131-6: 2002.

7. Reimund E. 'The free radical flux theory of sleep', *Medical Hypotheses*, 43; 231-3: 1994.

8. Koopman C, Nouriani B, Erickson V, Anupindi R, Butler LD, Bachmann MH, Sephton SE, Spiegel D. 'Sleep disturbances in women with metastatic breast cancer', *Breast Journal*, 8; 362-70: 2002.

9. Josefson D. 'Working the 'graveyard' shift increases risk of colorectal cancer', *British Medical Journal*, 326; 1286: 2003.

10. Meier-Ewert H K, Ridker P M, Rifai N, Regan M M, Price N J, Dinges, Mullington JM. 'Effect of sleep loss on C-reactive protein, an inflammatory marker of cardiovascular risk.' *Journal of the American College of Cardiology*, 43; 678-83: 2004.

11. Ayas NT, White D P, Manson J E, Stampfer M J, Speizer F E. Malhotra A, Hu F B. 'A prospective study of sleep duration and coronary heart disease in women.' *Archives of Internal Medicine*, 163, 141: 2003.

12. Ayas NT, White DP, Al-Delaimy WK, Manson JE, Stampfer MJ, Speizer FE, Patel SP, Hu FB. 'A prospective study of self-reported sleep duration and incident diabetes in women', *Diabetes Care*, 26; 380-4: 2003.

13. Hall M, Baum A, Buysse DJ, Prigerson HG, Kupfer DJ, Reynolds CF. 'Sleep as a mediator of the stress-immune relationship', *Psychosomatic Medicine*, 60; 48-51: 1998.

14. Vandeputte M, der Weerd A. 'Sleep disorders and depressive feelings: a global survey with the Beck depression scale', *Sleep Medicine*, 4; 343-5: 2003.

15. Johns MW. 'New method for measuring daytime sleepiness: the Epworth sleepiness scale', *Sleep*, 14; 540-5: 1991.

16. Spiegel K. Leproult R, Van Cauter E. 'Impact of sleep debt on metabolic and endocrine function', *Lancet*, 354; 1435-9: 1999.

CHAPTER 3

1. Jamieson AO. 'Sleep and alcohol', http://www.sleepmed.com/sf1096.html.

2. Roehrs T, Roth T. 'Sleep, sleepiness and alcohol use', *Alcohol Research and Health*, 25; 101-9: 2001.

3. Yesavage JA, Leirer VO. 'Hangover effects on aircraft pilots 14 hours after alcohol ingestion: a preliminary report', *American Journal of Psychiatry*, 143; 1546-50: 1986.

4. Netzer NC, Eliasson AH, Strohl KP. 'Women with sleep apnea have lower levels of sex hormones', *Sleep & Breathing*, 7; 25-9: 2003.

5. Luboshitzky R, Aviv A, Hefetz A, Herer P, Shen-Orr Z, Lavie L, Lavie P. 'Decreased pituitary-gonadal secretion in men with obstructive sleep apnea', *Journal of Clinical Endocrinology & Metabolism*, 87, 3394-8: 2002.

6. Davidson TM. 'The great leap forward: the anatomic basis for the acquisition of speech and obstructive sleep apnea', *Medical Hypothesis*, 4; 184-94: 2003.

7. National Health and Medical Research Council, 'Obstructive sleep apnoea: now you can sleep easy', http://www.health.gov.aunhmrc/media/2000rel/sleep.htm.

8. Plotnikof AG, Quigley JM. 'Prevalence of severe hypovitaminosis D in patients with persistent, nonspecific musculoskeletal pain', *Mayo Clinic Proceedings*, 78; 1463-70: 2000.

9. Kovacs FM, Abraira V, Pena A, Martin-Rodriquez JG, Sanchez-Vera M, Ferrer E, Ruano D, Guillen P, Gestoso M, Muriel A, Zamora J, Gil del Real MT, Mufraggi N. 'Effect of firmness of mattress on chronic non-specific low-back pain: randomised double blind controlled multicentre trial', *Lancet*, 362; 1599-604: 2003.

10. Dickson PR. 'Effect of a fleecy wollen underlay on sleep.' *Medical Journal of Australia*, 140;87-9: 1984.

11. Steel GD, Callaway M, Suedfeld P, Palinkas L. 'Human sleep-wake cycles in the high Arctic: effects of unusual photoperiodicity in a natural setting', *Biological Rhythm Research*, 26; 582-92: 1995.

12. Mercola, J. 'Is sleep position really important in SIDS'? http://www.mercola.com/2003/mar19/sids.htm.

13. Johansson CE, Roehrs T, Schuh K, Warbasse L. 'The effect of cocaine on mood and sleep in cocaine-dependent males', *Experimental and Clinical Psychopharmacology*, 7; 338-8: 1999.

14. Kalant H. 'The pharmacology and toxicology of "ecstasy" (MDMA) and related drugs', *Canadian Medical Association Journal*, 165; 917-28: 2001.

15. Van Wijngaarden E, Savitz DA, Jianwen C, Loomis D. 'Exposure to electromagnetic fields and suicide in electric utility workers: a nested case-controlled study', *Western Journal of Medicine*, 173; 94-100: 2000.

16. Touitou Y, Lambrozo J, Camus F, Charbuy H. 'Magnetic fields and the melatonin hypothesis: a study of workers chronically exposed to 50-Hz magnetic fields', *American Journal of Physiology. Regulatory, Integrative and Comparative Physiology*, 284: R1529-35: 2003.

17. Pasche B, Erman M, Hayduk R, Mitler MM, Reite M, Higgs L, Kuster N, Rossel C, Dafri U, Amato D, Barbault A, Lebet JP.. 'Effects of low energy emission therapy in chronic psychophysiological insomnia', *Sleep*, 19; 327-336: 1996.

18. King A C, Oman R F, Brassinton G S, Bliwise D L, Haskell W L. 'Moderate-intensity exercise and self-rated quality of sleep in older adults. A randomized controlled trial', *Journal of the American Medical Association,* 277; 32-7: 1997.

19. Tworoger SS, Yasui Y, Vitiello MV, Schwartz RS, Ulrich CM. Aiello EJ, Irwin ML, Bowen D, Potter JD, McTiernan A. 'Effects of a yearlong moderate-intensity exercise and a stretching intervention on sleep quality in postmenopausal women', *Sleep*, 26; 830-6: 2003.

20. Li F, Fisher K J, Harmer P, Irbe D, Tearse, Weiumer C. 'Tai chi and self-rated quality of sleep and daytime sleepiness in older adults: a randomized controlled trial.' *Journal of the American Geriatric Society*, 52; 892-900: 2004.

21. Vgontzas AN, Bixler EO, Lin HM. Prolo P, Mastorakos G, Vela-Bueno A, Kales A, Chrousos GP. 'Chronic insomnia is associated with nyctohemeral activation of the hypothalamic-pituitary-adrenal axis: clinical implications', *Journal of Clinical Endocrinology & Metabolism*, 86; 3787-94: 2001.

22. Alvarez B, Dahlitz M, Vignau J, Parks JD. 'The delayed sleep phase syndrome: clinical and investigative findings in 14 patients', *Journal of Neurology, Neurosurgery and Psychiatry*, 55; 665-70: 1992.

23. Van Cauter E, Leproult R, Plat L. 'Age-related changes in slow wave sleep and REM sleep and relationship with growth hormone and cortisol levels in healthy men.' *Journal of the American Medical Association*, 284; 861-8: 2000.

24. Gambineri A, Pelusi C, Pasquali R. 'Testosterone levels in obese male patients with obstructive sleep apnea syndrome: relation to oxygen desaturation, body weight, fat distribution and the metabolic parameters.' *Journal of Endocrinological Investigation*, 26; 493-8: 2003.

25. Kreuger JM, Majde JA. 'Humoral links between sleep and the immune system.' *Annals of the New York Academy of Sciences*, 992; 9-20: 2003.

26. Marshall L, Born J. 'Brain-immune interactions in sleep.' *International Reviews of Neurobiology*, 52; 93-131: 2002.

27. Reddy AB, Field MD, Maywood ES, Hastings MH. 'Differential resynchronisation of circadian clock gene expression within the suprachiasmatic nuclei of mice subjected to experimental jet lag.' *The Journal of Neuroscience*, 22; 7326-30: 2002.

28. Reilly T. 'Travel: physiology, jet-lag strategies.' In: Enclyclopedia of Sports Medicine and Science, Fahey TD (Editor), Internet Society for Sport Science: http://sportsci.org. 12 July 1998.

29. Cardinall DP, Bortman GP, Liotta G, Perez Lloret S, Albornoz LE, Cutrera RA, Batista J, Orega Galla P. 'A multifactorial approach employing melatonin to accelerate resynchronization of sleep-wake cycle after a 12 time-zone westerly transmeridian flight in elite soccer athletes.' *Journal of Pineal Research*, 32; 41-6: 2002.

30. Monk TH, Kennedy KS, Rose LR, Linenger JM. 'Decreased human circadian pacemaker influence after 100 days in space: a case study.' *Psychosomatic Medicine*, 63; 881-5: 2001.

31. Mishima K, Okawa M, Shimizu T, Hishikawa Y. 'Diminished melatonin secretion in the elderly caused by insufficient environmental illumination.' *The Journal of Clinical Endocrinology & Metabolism*, 86; 129-34: 2001.

32. Ford-Martin P. 'Phototherapy' Gale Encyclopedia of Medicine. http://www.findarticles.com/cf_dls/g.2601/0010/260100159/pl/article.html

33. Garcia-Borreguero D, Larrosa O, Bravo M. 'Parkinson's disease and sleep.' *Sleep Medicine Reviews*, 7; 115-129: 2003.

34. Bliwise D L, 'Sleep disorders in Alzheimer's disease and other dementias.' *Clinical Cornerstone*, 6, S16-28: 2004.

35. Hartmann E, Russ D, Oldfield M, Sivan I, Cooper S. 'Who has nightmares: The personality of the lifelong nightmare sufferer.' *Archives of General Psychiatry*, 44: 49-56: 1987.

36. Schatzman M. 'The meaning of dreaming', *New Scientist*, 36-9; January 1987.

37. Megirian D, Dmochowski J, Farkas GA. "Mechanism controlling sleep organization of the obese Zucker rats." *Journal of Applied Physiology*, 84; 253-6: 1998.

38. Petrovsky N, Harrison LC. 'The chronobiology of human cytokine production', *International Review of Immunology*, 16; 635-49: 1998.

39. Science Daily News Release, 15 February 2002. 'Dog Tired? It could be your pooch.' http://www.sciencedaily.com/ releases/22002/02/020215070932.htm

40. Rijnbeek B, de Visser SJ, Franson KL, Cohen AF, van Gerven JM. 'REM sleep effects as a biomarker for the effects of antidepressants in healthy volunteers.' *Journal of Psychopharmacology*, 17; 196-203: 2003.

41. Landolt HP, Kelsoe JR, Rapaport MH, Gillin JC. 'Rapid tryptophan depletion reverses phenellzine-induced suppression of REM sleep.' *Journal of Sleep Research*, 12; 13-8: 2003.

42. Djeridane Y, Touitou Y. 'Chronic diazepam administration differentially affects melatonin synthesis in rat pineal and Harderian glands.' *Psychopharmacology* (Berlin), 154; 403-7: 2001.

43. Horowitz TS, Cade BE, Wolfe JM, Czeisler CA. 'Efficacy of bright light and sleep/darkness scheduling in alleviating circadian maladaption to night work.' *American Journal of Physiology, Endocrinology and Metabolism*, 281; 384-91: 2001.

44. Wright SW, Lawrence LM, Wrenn KD, Haynes ML, Welch LW, Schlack HM. 'Randomized clinical trial of melatonin after night-shift work: efficacy and neuropsychologic effects.' *Annals of Emergency Medicine*, 32; 334-40: 1998.

45. Tuladhar R, Harding R, Cranage SM, Adamson TM, Horne RS. 'Effects of sleep position, sleep state and age on heart rate responses following provoked arousal in term infants.' *Early Human Development*, 71; 157-69: 2003.

46. Stepanski EJ, Wyatt JK. 'Use of sleep hygiene in the treatment of insomnia.' *Sleep Medicine Reviews*, 7; 215-25: 2003.

47. Lushington K, Dawson D, Lack I. 'Core body temperature is elevated during constant wakefulness in elderly poor sleepers.' *Sleep*, 23; 504-10: 2000.

48. Lushington K, Pollard K, Lack L, Kennaway DJ, Dawson D. 'Daytime melatonin administration in elderly good and poor sleepers: effects on core body temperature and sleep latency.' *Sleep*, 20; 1135-44: 1998.

49. Davis MDP, Sandroni P, Rooke TW, Low PA. 'Erythromelalgia: vasculopathy, neuropathy, or both?' *Archives of Dermatology*, 139; 1337-43: 2003.

50. Krauchi K, Cajochen C, Werth E, Wirz-Justice A. 'Warm feet promotes the rapid onset of sleep.' *Nature*, 401; 36-7: 1999.

51. Angus RG, Pearce DG, Buguet, Olsen L. 'Vigilance performance of men sleeping under arctic conditions.' *Aviation, Space and Environmental Medicine*, 50; 692-6: 1979.

52. Harvey AG, Payne S. 'The management of unwanted pre-sleep thoughts in insomnia: distraction with imagery versus general distraction.' *Behavior Research and Therapy*; 40; 267-77: 2002., '

53. Mason J, et al. Client centered hypnotherapy for tinnitus: who is likely to benefit?' *American Journal of Clinical Hypnotherapy*, 37; 294-9: 1995

54. Podoshin L, et al. Idiopathic subjective tinnitus treated by biofeedback, acupuncture and drug therapy. *Ear, Nose and Throat Journal,* 70; 284-9: 1991

55. Shemesh Z, et al. 'Vitamin B12 deficiency in patients with chronic tinnitus and noise-induced hearing loss.' *American Journal of Otolaryngology*, 14; 94-9: 1993

CHAPTER 4

1. Blumenthal M, Senior Editor. *The Complete German Commission E Monographs*, American Botanical Council, Austin, Texas, 1992.

2. Bensky, D; Gamble, A with T. Kaptchuk. 1993. *Chinese Herbal Medicine Materia Medica- revised edition*. Eastland Press. P 404- 405.

3. Phytotherapies. Org. 2000. *Monograph: Ziziphus spinosa*. http://www. phytotherapies.org/monograph_detail.cfm?id=246.

4. Dharmananda, S. 2001. *Ziziphus*. http://www.itmonline.org/arts/ ziziphus. htm.

5.Mills, S and Bone, K. 2005. *The Essential Guide to Herbal Safety*. Elsevier Churchill Livingstone. P 644- 645.

6. Akhondzadeh, S, Naghavi, HR, Vazirian M, Shayeganopour A, Rashidi H, Khani M. 'Passionflower in the treatment of generalized anxiety: a pilot double-blind randomized controlled trial with oxazepam.' *Journal of Clinical Pharmacy &Therapeutics*, 26; 363-7: 2001.

7. Rasmussen P. 'A role for phytotherapy in the treatment of benzodiazepine and opiate drug withdrawal.' *The European Journal of Herbal Medicine*, 3; 11: 1997.

8. Lehmann E, Kinzler E, Friedemann J. 'Efficacy of a special kava extract (*Piper methysticum*) in patients with states of anxiety, tension and excitedness of non-mental origin — double blind placebo controlled study of four weeks treatment.' *Phytomedicine*, 3; 113-9: 1996.

9. Munte TF, Heinze HJ, Matzke M. 'Effects of oxazepam and an extract of kava roots (Piper methysticum) on event related potentials in a word recognition task.' *Pharmacoelectroencephalog*, 27; 46-53: 1993.

10. Warnecke G. 'Psychosomatic dysfunction in the female climacteric. Clinical effectiveness and tolerance of kava extract WS 1490.' *Fortschritte der Medizin*, 109, 119-22, 1991.

11. Brown D, Reviewer. 'Standardised kava extract: clinical monograph.'*Quarterly Review of Natural Medicine*, Winter, 287-92: 1998.

12. Pittler MH, Ernst E. 'Efficacy of kava extract for treating anxiety: systematic review and meta-analysis.' *Journal of Clinical Psychopharmacology*, 20; 84-9: 2000.

13. Wheatley D. 'Stress-induced insomnia treated with kava and valerian: singly and in combination.' *Human Psychopharmacology*, 16; 353-6: 2001.

14. Complementary Medicines Evaluation Committee, Meeting 41, 1 August 2003. 'Safety Review of kava'. http://www.tgw.gov.au/docs/html/cmec/ cmecdr41.htm

15. Blumenthal, M (ed). *The Complete German Commission E Monographs*, American Botanical Council, Austin, Texas, 1998.

16. Donath F, Quispe S, Diefenbach K, Maurer A, Fietze I, Roots I. 'Critical evaluation of the effect of valerian extract on sleep structure and sleep quality.' *Pharmacopsychiatry*, 33; 47-53: 2000.

17. Herrera-Arellano A, Luna-Villegas G, Cuevas-Uriostegiu L, Alvarez L, Vargas-Pineda G, Zamilpa-Alvarez A, Tortoriello J. 'Polysomnographic evaluation of the hypnotic effect of Valeriana edulis standardized extract in patients suffering from insomnia.' *Planta Medica*, 67; 695-99: 2001.

18. Willey, LB. 'Valerian overdose: a case report.' *Veterinary and Human Tooxicology*, 37; 364-5: 1995.

19. Dressing H, Köhler S. Müller WE. 'Improvement of sleep quality with a high-dose valerian/lemon balm preparation.' *Psychopharmakotherapie*, 3: 123-40: 1996.

20. Hypericum Depression Trial Study Group. 'Effect of *Hypericum perforatum* (St John's wort) in major depressive disorder.' *Journal of the American Medical Association*, 287; 1807-14: 2002.

21. Blumenthal M, Senior Editor, *The Complete German Commission E Monographs*, American Botanical Council, Austin, Texas, 1998.

22. Gould L, Reddy CV, Gomprecht RF. 'Cardiac effects of chamomile tea.' *Journal of Clinical Pharmacology*, 13; 475-9: 1973.

23. Roberts A, Williams JM. 'The effect of olfactory stimulation on fluency, vividness of imagery and associated mood: a preliminary study.' *British Journal of Medical Psychology*, 65; 197-9: 1992.

CHAPTER 5

1. Tomoda A, Mike T, Matsukura M. 'Circadian rhythm abnormalities in adrenoleukodystrophy and methyl B12 treatment.' *Brain and Development*, 17; 428-31: 1995.

2. Yehuda S, Rabinovitz S, Mostofsky DI. 'Essential fatty acids and sleep: mini-review and hypothesis'. *Medical Hjypotheses*, 50; 139-45: 1998.

3. Held K, Antonijevic IA, Kunzel H, Uhr M, Wetter TC, Golly IC, Steiger A, Murck, H. 'Oral Mg (2+) supplementation reverses age-related neuroendocrine and sleep EEG changes in humans.' *Pharmacopsychiatry*, 35: 135-43: 2002.

4. Boeve BF, Silber MH, Ferman TH. 'Melatonin for treatment of REM sleep behavior disorder in neurologic disorders: results in 14 patients.' *Sleep Medicine*, 4; 281-4: 2003.

5. Zhdanova IV, Wurtman RJ, Regan MM, Taylor JA, Shi JP, Leclair OU. 'Melatonin treatment for age-related insomnia.' *The Journal of Clinical Endocrinology & Metabolism*, 86; 4727-30: 2001.

6. Garfinkel D, Zisapel N, Wainstein J, Landon M. 'Facilitation of benzodiazepine discontinuation by melatonin.' *Archives of Internal Medicine*, 159; 2456-60: 1999.

7. Lockley SW, Skene DJ, Arendt J, Tabandeh H, Bird AC, Defrance R. 'Relationship between melatonin rhythms and visual loss in the blind.' *Journal of Clinical Endocrinology & Metabolism*, 82; 3763-70: 1997.

8. Foscher S, Smolnik R, Herms M, Born J, Fehm HL. 'Melatonin acutely improves the neuroendocrine architecture of sleep in blind individuals.' *The Journal of Clinical Endocrinology & Metabolism*, 88; 5315-20: 2003.

9. Reiter RH. 'Melatonin: clinical relevance.' *Best Practice & Research: Clinical Endocrinology & Metabolism*, 17; 273-85: 2003.

10. Thomas VCR, Reiter RJ, Herman TS. 'Melatonin: from basic research to cancer treatment.' *Journal of Clinical Oncology*, 20; 2575-2601: 2002.

11. Hersheimer A, Waterhouse J. 'The prevention and treatment of jeg lag.' *British Medical Journal*, 326; 296-7: 2003.

12. Sheldon SH. 'Pro-convulsant effects of oral melatonin in neurologically disabled children.' *Lancet*, 351; 1254: 1998.

13. National Institute of Neurological Disorders and Stroke. "Brain basics: understanding sleep." http://www.ninds.nih.gov/health_and_medical/pubs/ understanding_sleep_brain_basic_.htm.

14. Gutierrez CI, Urbina M, Obregion F, Glykys J, Lima L. 'Characterization of tryptophan high affinity transport system in pinealocytes of the rat. Day-night modulation.' *Amino acids*, 25; 95-105: 2003.

15. Lindsley JG, Hartmann EL, Mitchell W. 'Selectivity in response to L-tryptophan among insomniac subjects: a preliminary report.' *Sleep*, 6; 247-56: 1983.

16. Lin Y. 'Acupuncture treatment for insomnia and acupuncture analgesia.' *Psychiatry and Clinical Neuroscience*, 49; 119-20: 1995.

17. Editorial, 'Sensory stimulation in dementia.' *British Medical Journal*, 325; 1312-13: 2002.

18. Hardy M, Kirk-Smith ME, Stretch DD. 'Replacement of drug treatment for insomnia by ambient odor.' *Lancet*, 346: 701: 1995.

19. Ghelardini C, Galeotti N, Salvatore G, Mazzanti G. 'Local anaesthetic activity of the essential oil of Lavandula angustifolia.' *Planta Medica*, 63: 700-3: 1999.

20. Kagawa D, Jokura H, Ochial R, Tokimitsu I, Tsubone H. 'The sedative effects and mechanism of action of cedrol inhalation with behavioral pharmacological evaluation.' *Planta Medica*, 69; 637-41: 2003.

21. Dorsey CM, Teicher MH, Cohen-Zion M, Stefanovic L, Satlin A, Tartarini W, Harper D, Lukas SE. 'Core body temperature and sleep of older female insomniacs before and after passive body heating.' *Sleep*, 22; 891-8: 1999.

22. Sung EJ, Tochihara Y. 'Effects of bathing and hot footbath on sleep in winter.' *Journal of Physiological Anthropology and Applied Human Science*, 19; 21-7: 2000.

23. Murphy PJ, Campbell SS. 'Nighttime drop in body temperature: a physiological trigger for sleep onset.' *Sleep*, 20; 505-11: 1997.

24. Edinger J D, Duke University Medical Center, 'Behavioral therapy effective in treatment of insomnia.' 10 April 2001. http://www.dukenews.duke.edu/Med/sleep1.htm

25. Davidson RJ, Kabat-Zinn J, Schumacher J, Rosenkranz M, Muller D, Santorelli SF, Urbanowski F, Harrington A, Bonus K, Sheridan JF. 'Alterations in brain and immune function produced by mindfulness meditation.' *Psychosomatic Medicine*, 65; 564-70: 2003.

26. Khare KC, Nigam SK. 'A study of electroencephalogram in meditators.' *Indian Journal of Physiology and Pharmacology*, 33; 173-8: 2000.

27. Horohov DW, Pourclau SS, Mistric L, Chapman A, Ryan DH. 'Increased dietary fat prevents sleep deprivation-induced immune suppression in rats.' *Complementary Medicine*, 51; 230-3: 2001.

28. Hattori A, Migitake H, ligo M, Itoh M, Yamamoto K, Ohtani-Kaneko R, Hara M, Suzuki T, Reiter RJ. 'Identification of melatonin in plants and its effects on plasma melatonin levels and binding to melatonin receptors in vertebrates.' *Biochemistry and Molecular Biology International*, 35; 627-34: 1995.

29. Burkhardt S, Tan DX, Manchester LC, Hardeland R, Reiter RJ. 'Detection and quantification of the antioxidant melatonin in Montmorency and Balaton tart cherries (Prunis cerasus)'. *Journal of Agriculture and Food Chemistry*, 49; 4898-3900: 2001.

APPENDIX IV

1. Ray Nimmo, "Benzodiazepine addiction, withdrawal and recovery". http://www.benzo.org.uk

2. Morin CM, Bastien C, Guay B, Radouco-Thomas M, Leblanc J, Vallieres A. 'Randomized clinical trial of supervised tapering and cognitive behavior therapy to facilitate benzodiazepine discontinuation in older adults with chronic insomnia.' *American Journal of Psychiatry*, 161; 332-42: 2004.

APPENDIX V

1. Lockley SW, Skene DJ, Arendt J, Tabandeh H, Bird AC, Defrance R. 'Relationship between melatonin rhythms and visual loss in the blind.' *Journal of Clinical Endocrinology & Metabolism*, 82; 3763-70: 1997.

2. Foscher S, Smolnik R, Herms M, Born J, Fehm HL. 'Melatonin acutely improves the neuroendocrine architecture of sleep in blind individuals.' *The Journal of Clinical Endocrinology & Metabolism*, 88; 5315-20: 2003.

3. Cartwright RD. 'The role of sleep in changing our minds: A psychologist's discussion of papers on memory reactivation and consolidation in sleep.' *Learning & Memory*, 11; 660-3: 2004

INDEX

B

C

D

E

F

G

Infertility:
the hidden causes

In this well researched book, Dr Sandra Cabot and naturopath Margaret Jasinska explore the many hidden causes of infertility which are often easily overcome.

One in six couples experience infertility. They are often left confused, hopeless and with no definitive answers as to what can be done to improve their chance of conceiving. Infertility is not a disease; rather it is a symptom of an underlying health problem.

By improving the health of both prospective parents, not only will this dramatically increase the chance of achieving a healthy pregnancy; it will also increase the likelihood of having a healthy baby.

In this book Dr Sandra Cabot and naturopath Margaret Jasinska help you to overcome problems that compromise fertility, such as:

- Endometriosis
- Balance your hormones naturally
- Overcome polycystic ovarian syndrome
- Overcome immune system disorders
- Reduce exposure to environmental chemicals
- Overcome hidden infections
- Vitamin and/or mineral deficiencies
- Understand tests you must have when trying to conceive

- Identify and overcome factors that lead to male infertility
- Increase sperm counts and improve the quality of sperm
- Improve your chance of success with IVF
- Maintain a healthy pregnancy
- Reduce the risk of miscarriage
- Give your baby the best possible start in life

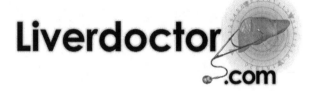

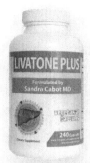

I am so glad I have been able to assist thousands of people to regain their health and vitality.

Sandra Cabot

Dr Sandra Cabot MBBS DRCOG

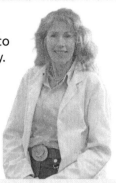

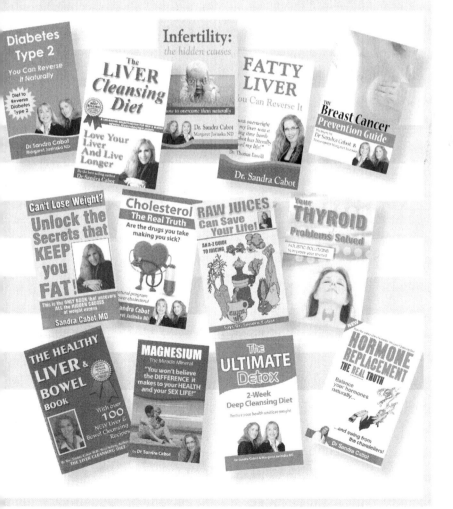

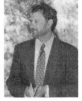